Gastric Bypass Cookbook

100+ Quick and Easy Recipes for stage 1 and 2 After Gastric Bypass Surgery

Bonus:
FREE Report Reveals The Secrets To Lose Weight

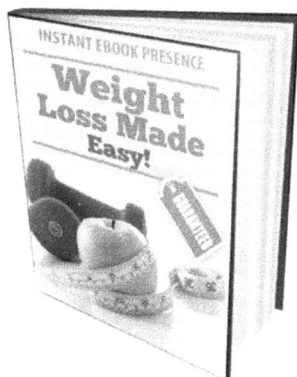

Weight loss doesn't happen from dieting only. Diets are short term solutions to shed extra weight. Diets do not work in the long term because people hate being on a diet (it's ok, you can admit that here). The only long term solution for permanent weight loss is to create new eating habits. This doesn't mean that chocolate will never pass your lips again, but it does mean looking after yourself and watching what you eat...

You can lose weight when you have the right reasons and motivation, and a part of this guide is to help you to find the motivation you need to change your weight...

Go to Get This Guid For FREE

http://www.sportsforsoul.com/weight-loss-2/

Table of Contents

Snacks and Appetizers 99

Introduction

Congratulations on downloading your personal copy of *Gastric Bypass Cookbook.* Thank you for doing so.

The following chapters will provide you with many recipes to help you through your gastric bypass diet.

There are plenty of books on this subject on the market, thanks again for choosing this one! Every effort was made to ensure it is full of as much useful information as possible. Please enjoy!

Congratulations on downloading your personal copy of *Gastric Bypass Cookbook*. Thank you for doing so.

Breakfast

Fried Egg on Parmesan Toast

Ingredients

Halved baby tomatoes – optional

Salad leaves – optional

Pepper

Salt

Egg

¼ c parmesan cheese, grated

Instructions

Warm your skillet to a very high heat. Test by dropping some water in the pan, it should sizzle as soon as it hits the pan. It needs to be this hot for this to come out correctly.

Place the cheese in an even layer and spread out so that it is larger than a fried egg. Continue to cook until the cheese starts to bubble up. This shouldn't take but 30 to 50 seconds.

Crack your egg on the cheese. Let the egg cook until the edges have set, this takes about two minutes. Place a lid over the pan and let it continue to cook until the egg has cooked to your liking. The cheese should also be crisped and golden.

Add pepper and salt to your egg. Carefully run a spatula around the cheese and loosen it up. Lift it out and onto a plate.

You can serve with tomatoes and salad leaves if you would like or with your favorite breakfast meats.

Pumpkin Pie Oatmeal

Ingredients

1 scoop vanilla protein powder

¼ c water

Sweetener of choice to taste

2 tbsp oven roasted sliced almonds

¼ c canned pumpkin

Pinch nutmeg

Pinch cinnamon

½ c old fashioned oats

¾ c water

½ c nonfat milk

Instructions

Let some water come up to a boil. Place in nutmeg, cinnamon, and oatmeal. Cook until liquid is gone. Stir occasionally.

When liquid is gone, stir in sweetener, almonds, pumpkin. Set to the side.

Combine protein powder and water in a different bowl. Mix until powder is dissolved, you might have to use a blender.

Pour protein mix over oatmeal and serve.

BBQ Chicken Breakfast Burritos

Ingredients

½ oz 2% sharp cheddar cheese

Dash of salt

1 tbsp barbecue sauce

1 tsp cumin

1 tsp garlic

2 low-fat tortillas

4 oz chicken breast

4 egg whites

Instructions

Scramble the egg whites in a pan sprayed with Pam. Add salt, garlic, and cumin. Stir until the desired doneness. Put half of the chicken breast into a tortilla. Add ½ of the cheese, ½ of the barbecue sauce, and you can add hot sauce if desired. Add half the egg on top. You can add cilantro, onions, and tomatoes if desired. Roll into burritos and serve.

Very Berry Smoothie

Ingredients

½ c nonfat yogurt

½ c nonfat milk

½ c ice

½ c frozen strawberries

½ c frozen blueberries

Instructions

Place all of the above into your blender. Mix until creamy and smooth. Enjoy.

Ricotta Muffins

Ingredients

4 large eggs

2 to 3 tsp Splenda

2 tsp vanilla extract

2 c ricotta cheese

Instructions

Your oven should be at 400. Fill a regular muffin tin with liners. Spray the liners with some nonstick spray.

Stir together all ingredients until smooth. Pour into muffin cups.

Bake 20 to 30 minutes. It will be done when a toothpick inserted comes out clean.

Feel free to add fresh blueberries or blackberries before baking. These freeze great.

Baked Oatmeal

Ingredients

2 tbsp unsalted slivered almonds

1/3 c craisins

1 tsp vanilla

1 ½ tsp cinnamon

4 tsp Splenda brown sugar

½ c unsweetened applesauce

2 large eggs

1/3 c Splenda

1 c low-fat buttermilk

½ tsp salt

1 ½ tsp baking powder

2 c quick cooking oats

Instructions

Your oven should be at 325. Coat a pie plate with nonstick spray.

Take the dry ingredients and mix them together. Place in the wet and mix well. Place this into your pie plate.

Place in the oven for 40 to 45 minutes. Take out of the oven. Let cool. Cut into 8 equal servings. Store in refrigerator or freezer.

This is the consistency of coffee cake but very good for you. Can be eaten as breakfast, snack, or dessert.

Egg Cups

Ingredients

Pepper

Salt

1 tbsp chopped chives

½ c 2% shredded cheddar cheese

6 eggs

6 slices lean deli ham

Instructions

Your oven should be at 350. Coat a six cups in a muffin pan with nonstick spray.

Arrange ham slices to line the muffin cups. The edges might stick up some, that is fine. Bake for 10 minutes. Take out of the oven. Break an egg into each cup. Break the yolks gently. Sprinkle with pepper and salt.

Put back in for another ten minutes. Check the eggs, if they are to your liking remove, sprinkle with chives and cheese. Enjoy.

If they aren't to your liking, continue to cook. Check each minute.

Broccoli Quiche

Ingredients

½ c canned mushrooms

¼ c fat-free half and half

1 large head broccoli

3 oz. low-fat Swiss cheese

¼ c skim milk

1 c egg substitute

Instructions

Your oven should be at 400. A pie plate should be greased with some nonstick spray.

Steam broccoli. Chop.

Add mushrooms and broccoli to pie plate.

Combine half and half, skim milk, and egg substitute. Mix well.

Pour over mushrooms and broccoli. Sprinkle with cheese.

Bake about 40 minutes.

Cut into four equal servings and enjoy.

Breakfast Popsicles

Ingredients

1 cup mixed berries or chopped fruit of choice

½ c oats

½ c 1% milk

1 c Greek yogurt

Instructions

Mix yogurt and milk. Equally, divide mixture into popsicle molds. Put some berries in each. Equally, divide the oatmeal into each mold. Put a wooden stick into each mold and put in the freezer. Freeze a minimum of four hours before eating. If popsicles won't unmold easily. Run under warm water for a few seconds.

PB&J Pancakes

Ingredients

1 c frozen mixed berry blend

4 large egg whites

2 tbsp powdered peanuts

½ c instant oatmeal

½ c low-fat cottage cheese

Instructions

There is a certain order in which these should be placed into the blender. The first ingredient is cottage cheese. The second ingredient should be oatmeal. The third ingredient should be powdered peanuts. The last ingredient will be egg whites. Blend until smooth and pancake batter. Pour into a bowl and add fruit mix. Spray skillet with cooking spray. Makes four to seven pancakes according to size.

Pumpkin Pie Oatmeal

Ingredients

½ c no salt added 1% cottage cheese

1 tsp Truvia

Dash ground ginger

Dash ground cloves

1/8 tsp cinnamon

½ c canned pumpkin

1/3 c old fashioned oats

Instructions

Mix sweetener, spices, pumpkin, and oats in a microwavable bowl. Microwave on high 90 seconds. Stir in cottage cheese. Microwave another 60 seconds. Wait 2 minutes before eating.

Egg Burrito

Ingredients

2 tbsp salsa

1 oz protein of choices like ground beef, chicken, or tofu

1 tbsp shredded Mexican blend cheese

Salt

2 tbsp. plain fat-free Greek yogurt

Pepper

1 egg + 1 egg white

Instructions

Put egg white and egg in small bowl. Beat well. Spray skillet with cooking spray. When hot, pour eggs into heated pan. Spread to coat pan. Let eggs set to allow edges to set. Sprinkle them with pepper and salt. Flip over.

Let the other side cook until completely cooked. Put on a plate. In the center of the egg, add cheese, and protein of choice. Roll up egg to form a burrito. Add Greek yogurt and salsa if desired.

Cottage Cheese Pancakes

Ingredients

3 eggs, lightly beaten

½ tbsp. canola oil

1 c low-fat cottage cheese

½ tsp baking soda

1/3 c all-purpose flour

Instructions

Sift baking soda and flour in small bowl.

Mix rest of the ingredients in large bowl.

Pour flour into wet ingredients and stir to incorporate.

Spray skillet with nonstick spray. Once everything is hot, place 1/3 cup batter in your hot skillet and cook until bubble starts to form on the top. Flip and cook brown another side.

Serve with low-calorie syrup.

Egg Muffin

Ingredients

¼ tsp Italian seasoning

¼ tsp salt

¼ tsp pepper

½ c 1% milk

¾ c shredded low-fat shredded cheese of choice

12 slices turkey bacon

6 large eggs

Instructions

Spray muffin pan with cooking spray. Heat oven to 350.

Put three slices of bacon in bottom of every muffin cup.

Mix all other ingredients together until well mixed. Save ¼ cup shredded cheese. Put ¼ cup of egg mixture in each cup. Sprinkle a bit more cheese over them.

Bake around 25 minutes. The eggs should be set.

Cheese Spiced Pancakes

Ingredients

Pancakes:
Low-fat cooking spray
1 tbsp sugar or artificial sweetener
Pinch salt
½ c AP flour
3 eggs, separated
1 tsp mixed spice, ground
8 oz spreadable goat cheese
Option Adult Toppings:
1 measure brandy
2 oz cranberries
Sweetener

4 tangerines, peeled

Instructions

For making the pancakes, combine the egg yolks, mixed spice, and the cheese. Then beat in the salt and the flour.

Beat the whites of the eggs until they become stiff then whisk in your sweetener of choice. Fold this into the cheese.

If you are making the optional topping, put the sweetener and tangerines in a pan. Stir occasionally until your tangerines start to release their juices and it starts looking a little syrupy. Mix in the brandy and cranberries. Place it to the side until it's time to use it.

Add a bit of cooking spray to your skillet. Let it heat up and add three large spoonfuls of your batter into your pan. Let it cook for two minutes, or the edges form bubbles. Flip the pancake and cook until done. Take out and continue. The batter should make 12 pancakes.

Divide up the pancakes between four different plates spoon the topping over them.

Flour-Less Pancakes

Ingredients

Low-fat spray

Milk to mix

1 banana

1 egg

1 c rolled oats

Instructions

Put the banana, oats, and egg into your food processor and mix it up until it is smooth. Add a bit of milk and blend. Continue adding mix until your mixture reaches a slightly runny consistency. Three tablespoons should be able to help.

Let this mixture sit for around 15 minutes; this will allow the mixture to thicken up a bit.

Spritz some of the cooking spray onto a skillet. Let it heat up and a spoonful of the mixture to make a medallion sized pancake. Place as many on your pan as you can as long as you still have room to flip them. Let the first side cook for a minute and then flip, cooking another minute. Keep the pancakes warm as you finish up your batter.

Serve the pancakes with sugar-free syrup, yogurt, and fruit, or a dust of sugar with a drizzle of lemon. You can also enjoy them plain.

Chocolate Porridge

Ingredients

Sugar-free syrup

Chopped fruits, nuts, or seeds

1 square dark chocolate, unsweetened – optional

1 tbsp cocoa powder

4 tbsp porridge oats

1 c milk, skim

Instructions

Put the chocolate, if using, cocoa powder, oats, and milk into a microwavable bowl.

Heat this in the microwave for two minutes. Mix everything and then cook for another 15 to 20 seconds.

Place in a severing bowl and then add your desired toppings on top.

Ham and Egg Roll Up

Ingredients

20 ham slices

1 c tomatoes, chopped

1 ½ c cheddar cheese, shredded

2 tbsp butter

1 c baby spinach

Pepper

Salt

2 tsp garlic powder

10 eggs

Instructions

Heat up your broiler. Crack the eggs into a bowl and whisk them with the pepper, salt, and garlic powder.

In a skillet, place in the butter and let it melt. Pour in the eggs and scramble them until they are done. Mix in the cheddar, and stir until melted. Fold in the tomatoes and the spinach.

Place two pieces of ham on a cutting board. Add a spoonful of eggs, and then roll it up. Continue until you use up the ham and the eggs.

Put the roll-ups in a baking dish and broil five minutes.

Bunless Breakfast Sandwich

Ingredients

½ avocado, mashed

¼ c cheddar cheese, shredded

2 tbsp water

2 slices bacon, cooked

2 eggs

Instructions

Put two mason jar lids into your skillet and spray the pan with nonstick spray and allow it to heat up. Crack an egg into each of the lids and whisk the egg slightly just to break up the yolks.

Pour some water into the pan and place a lid over the skillet. Let this cook and steam the egg whites. Let this cook for three minutes. Take the lid off and place the cheese on one of the eggs. Let it cook until the cheese has become melty, around a minute.

Place the egg bun that doesn't have the cheese on a plate. Place on the avocado and the bacon. Lay the other egg bun with the cheese side down on top. Enjoy.

Main Dishes

Lamb Souvlaki

Ingredients

16 cherry tomatoes
1 garlic clove, crushed
1 tsp oregano – or ½ tsp dried oregano
2 yellow peppers, cored sliced into bite-sized pieces
12 oz lean lamb, cubed – 12 to 16 pieces
Pepper
1 red onion, sliced into eight wedges
Salt
1 tbsp EVOO
Sauce:
1 tbsp lemon juice
8 oz plain yogurt, low-fat
1 garlic clove, crushed

2 cucumbers, peeled, chopped finely, and drained

Instructions

Stir the pepper, oregano, salt, garlic, and olive oil together. Taste and adjust any of the seasonings that you need to. This is the marinade for your lamb.

Slide the tomatoes, onion, pepper, and lamb onto four different skewers, alternating them, and lay them into a shallow dish. Brush them with the marinade, place a covering over them, and then refrigerate. They should chill for at least two to three hours for the best flavor. When you can, turn them and brush with extra marinade.

You can grill or bake the skewers for five to eight minutes or until the lamb has cooked to medium and are slightly charred. If you want them more well done, cook a little longer.

As they cook, mix together the pepper, garlic, salt, yogurt, lemon juice, and cucumber for your sauce. Serve the sauce along side of the skewers and a slice of pita bread.

Chicken Parmesan

Ingredients

Pepper

Salt

3 tbsp parmesan cheese

½ c hard cheese, low-fat and grated

1 c tomato pasta sauce

1 lb chicken breast fillets, skinless

Instructions

Your oven should be set to 375.

The chicken should be placed in your casserole dish and put the tomato sauce over it.

Add the pepper, salt, parmesan, and the grated hard cheese.

Put this for 25 to 30 minutes in the oven. Make sure the chicken is at 160

This can be served with roasted veggies, pasta, rice, baked potato, or a salad.

Turkey Soup

Ingredients

Salt

Pepper

½ tsp garlic powder

3 cans diced tomatoes

3 tbsp chicken bouillon granules

8 c water

10 oz bag frozen mixed veggies

1 pound ground turkey

1 large zucchini, chopped

2 stalks chopped celery

10 oz mushrooms, sliced

1 large chopped onion

1 tbsp olive oil

Instructions

Sauté zucchini, mushrooms, and onions in pan until soft.

Add ground turkey. Cook until browned.

Put into crockpot. Add remaining ingredients. Place in water. Place on the lid and set on low for six to eight hours.

This recipe freezes well. You may substitute favorite vegetables as you like.

Unstuffed Green Peppers

Ingredients

½ c rice

½ tsp basil

1 tsp garlic powder

1 large diced onion

2 large diced green peppers

2 large diced tomatoes

1 lb lean ground beef

Instructions

Cook half cup rice with 1 cup water per package directions.

Brown ground beef in skillet. Drain. Spoon onto paper towels to drain completely.

Put onion, basil, garlic powder, green peppers, and tomatoes. Let this cook for 15 minutes. Place in cooked rice and ground beef. Stir to combine. Add pepper and salt to taste.

Serve and enjoy.

Italian Chicken

Ingredients

2 lbs skinless, boneless chicken breast

3 c cooked long grain rice

½ c water

1 packet Italian dressing mix

1 can fat-free cream of chicken soup

1 package reduced fat cream cheese

Instructions

Put chicken in your slow cooker.

Combine the water with the dressing mix until well combined. Place this on the chicken.

Place on the lid. Set to low for 8 hours.

Mix the soup and cream cheese together in a bowl.

Set the chicken aside. Shred with two forks.

Pour soup mixture into crock pot and stir to combine.

Put chicken back into crock pot. Stir to combine. Let it continue to cook until everything has heated through.

Serve alongside rice.

Mexican Chicken

Ingredients

¼ c light sour cream

1 ½ tsp taco seasoning

½ can cheddar cheese soup

½ c salsa

1 skinless, boneless chicken breast cut in half

Instructions

Put chicken in slow cooker. Sprinkle taco seasoning over chicken. Stir cheese soup and salsa together and place it over the chicken. Cover. Set for eight hours on low.

Take the chicken out from slow cooker and shred. Put it back in the cooker and mix together. Add sour cream and stir again.

This can be served over rice or used as taco, burrito, or enchilada filling.

Shrimp Ceviche

Ingredients

1 small finely diced red onion

2 serrano chili, seeds and ribs removed, diced

1 bunch cilantro, chopped finely

1 lb medium raw shrimp, peeled and deveined

4 medium tomatoes, diced

1 cup lime juice

Instructions

Combine lime juice and shrimp in a bowl. Place a lid over it and marinate for 15 minutes or until they turn pink. Don't marinate too long. It will make the shrimp tough.

Add cilantro, chili peppers, tomatoes, and onions.

Stir to combine. Season with pepper and salt.

Serve and enjoy.

Chicken Caprese

Ingredients

1 tbsp olive oil

Pepper

1 lb boneless, skinless chicken breast

2 tbsp chopped basil

1 tsp Italian seasoning

3 tbsp balsamic vinegar

4 1 oz slices mozzarella cheese

4 ½-inch slices tomatoes

Instructions

Heat a grill pan or grill.

Place the olive oil on the chicken breasts. Sprinkle with pepper and salt. Sprinkle with Italian seasoning. Grill five minutes each side. Cooking time might vary due to the thickness of chicken.

When chicken is done, place mozzarella cheese on top and cook for another minute.

Remove and place on a plate.

Top with tomato, basil, and pepper.

Drizzle with balsamic vinegar. Serve and enjoy.

Chicken Parmesan

Ingredients

1 tbsp dried

1 tsp garlic powder

¼ c Italian bread crumbs

Crushed red pepper flakes

2 tbsp olive oil

12 oz chicken breast

1 tbsp Parmesan cheese, grated

Instructions

Heat oven to 365.

Filet the chicken breast in two separate pieces. Rub with olive oil.

Mix the above dry ingredients together. Coat each breast piece with dry mixture until well covered.

Bake 20 minutes.

Serve with favorite vegetables or spaghetti.

Salsa Chicken

Ingredients

1 package reduced sodium taco seasoning

½ c reduced fat sour cream

1 can reduced[-fat cream of mushroom soup

1 c salsa

4 skinless, boneless chicken breast

Instructions

Put chicken in slow cooker. Add in the taco seasoning. Place in the salsa. Put on the lid. Cook low for eight hours. Shred chicken. Place chicken back in cooker. Place in sour cream and stir well. Serve with rice.

Taco Stew

Ingredients

1 chopped onion

1 14.5 oz can diced tomatoes

1 15 oz can corn, drained

1 8 oz can tomato sauce

1 10.5 oz can diced tomatoes with chilies

1 15 oz can black beans

1 packet taco seasoning

1 to 2 boneless skinless chicken breast

1 15 oz can kidney beans

Instructions

Add everything to crock pot except chicken. Mix well. Put chicken on top. Place on a lid and cook for eight hours on low. 30 minutes before finished, take out chicken and shred. Put chicken back into cooker and stir.

Ladle into bowls. Serve with sour cream, cheese, sliced green onions, cilantro, or your favorite taco toppings, and tortilla chips.

Mexican Casserole

Ingredients

½ c shredded cheese

4 c water

1 15oz can black beans, drained and rinsed

2 c uncooked brown rice

1 10.75 oz can cheddar cheese soup

1 15.25 oz can sweet corn, undrained

1 diced small onion

1 diced green pepper

1 16 oz jar salsa

2 chicken breasts, boiled and shredded

Instructions

Heat oven to 400.

In large casserole dish, mix brown rice, corn, black beans, soup. Add water and mix thoroughly.

The onion and pepper should be cooked so that they are soft. Place in shredded chicken and heat through. Add this to the rice. Stir to combine well. Cover with lid or foil.

Bake 45 minutes. Stir occasionally. Carefully remove foil. Add a half cup of the cheese. Top with sour cream and tortilla chips.

Chili

Ingredients

2 tsp salt

1 14.5 oz can diced tomatoes

1 medium diced onion

2 14.5 oz cans kidney beans

1 14.5 oz can pureed tomatoes

8 oz chopped mushrooms

2 cloves minced garlic

3 tbsp chili powder

1 tbsp olive oil

1 lb lean ground beef

Instructions

Sauté mushrooms and onion in a pan with olive until soft. Add ground beef; breaking it up. Place in garlic, salt, chili powder, kidney beans, and tomatoes. Stir well to combine. Let it come to a boil. Turn to a simmer for about two hours.

Serve over rice with sour cream, shredded cheese, and avocado as toppings.

Pepper Steak

Ingredients

1 14.5 oz can diced tomatoes

1 can mushrooms

1 to 2 red bell peppers

1 medium chopped onions

¼ c salsa

1.5 to 2 lbs lean round steak, sliced into strips

Instructions

Put the above in your slow cooker. Place on the lid. Place on low. Cook 8 hours.

Serve with mashed potatoes or rice.

Sante Fe Soup

Ingredients

2 c water

2 11 oz. cans shoepeg corn, drained

1 large chopped onion

1 15 oz can kidney beans, undrained

2 14 oz. cans diced tomatoes, undrained

1 15 oz can pinto beans, undrained

1 envelope ranch dressing mix

1 10 oz. can tomatoes with green chilies, undrained

1 15 oz can black beans, undrained

2 envelopes taco seasoning

1 lb chicken breast, boiled and chopped

Instructions

Place the above in your slow cooker. Give a good stir. Cover. Set to low. Cook for four hours.

Beef and Gravy

Ingredients

½ tsp garlic powder

1 can 98% fat-free cream of mushroom soup

1 stalk diced celery

1 medium sliced onion

2 tbsp flour

1 lb stew beef

½ tsp pepper

Instructions

Place onion across the bottom of crock pot. Mix garlic, flour, and pepper in a bowl. Cover the meat with mixture. Put meat on top of onions. Pour soup over meat. Top with diced celery. Cover. Set to low. Cook eight hours.

Serve over rice or mashed potatoes.

Rainbow Trout

Ingredients

2 tsp olive oil

Pinch salt

¼ tsp pepper

¼ tsp celery seeds

1 1/3 tbsp chopped parsley

3 tbsp yellow cornmeal

8 oz. rainbow trout fillets

Instructions

Clean and rinse fish. Check for bones. Pat dry.

Mix parsley, celery seed, pepper, salt, and cornmeal.

Coat fish with mixture. Press to make sure it sticks.

Put olive oil in skillet. Cook a few minutes on each side. Fish will be brown and crispy. Should flake easily when pierced with a fork.

Creamy Spinach and Chicken Bake

Ingredients

1 c shredded Mozzarella

2 tsp garlic powder

¼ c Parmesan cheese

½ c fat-free sour cream

10 oz baby spinach

2 c diced cooked chicken breast

½ c light mayonnaise

Instructions

Your oven should be at 350. Coat a casserole dish with nonstick spray. Steam spinach, drain well. Mix garlic powder, cheese, mayonnaise, and sour cream. Pour half into casserole dish. Add chicken and spinach. Cover with remaining sour cream mixture. Bake 45 minutes until heated and bubbly.

Broiled Parmesan Tilapia

Ingredients

Salt

1 tsp chopped garlic

4 4 oz. tilapia filet

1 tbsp. lime juice

2 tbsp. grated parmesan cheese

½ tsp dried dill

1 tbsp light mayonnaise

Instructions

Heat oven to broil.

Put tilapia on broiling pan and sprinkle with salt and half of the dill. Put on the top rack and broil for three minutes. While broiling, mix the remaining ingredients. Don't forget the remaining dill. Take tilapia out of the oven, spread parmesan mixture over filets. Place in oven for three more minutes.

Creole Shrimp

Ingredients

4 c cook rice

1 ½ lbs peeled and deveined shrimp

6 c fat-free chicken broth

½ tsp thyme

½ tsp oregano

½ tsp red pepper flakes

6 tbsp tomato paste

2 medium chopped green bell pepper

4 chopped celery ribs

3 cloves minced garlic

2 medium chopped onions

2 tbsp olive oil

Instructions

Heat a pot with some oil. Place in garlic and all vegetables. Cook until soft. Place in thyme, red pepper flakes, oregano, and tomato paste. Cook until fragrant. Add broth and allow it to come to a boil. Cook until beginning to thicken around 30 minutes. Add shrimp and cook until opaque.

Serve over cooked rice.

Sweet Potato and Chicken Stew

Ingredients

Dash of oregano

Pinch of cumin

2 c 99% fat-free chicken broth

1 medium diced onion

1 ½ cups frozen corn

2 c fat-free salsa

1 large diced sweet potato

12 oz boneless skinless chicken breast, diced

Instructions

Put the above, except corn, into slow cooker. Cover. Set to low. Cook six hours. 30 minutes before done, add corn. Cook remaining 30 minutes.

Cola Chicken

Ingredients

1 c ketchup

3 boneless skinless chicken breast

1 12 oz can diet cola of choice

Instructions

Sear the chicken first in your pan. Pour cola and ketchup on top. Bring to boil. Cover. Simmer about 45 minutes. Uncover, bring back to a boil and boil until it thickens up and sticks to chicken. Watch the chicken carefully during this stage as it will burn.

Cranberry Chicken

Ingredients

Salt

Pepper

6 tsp Splenda

1 c fresh cranberries

2 5 oz chicken breast

Instructions

Put water, Splenda, and cranberries in a pot. Let it come to a boil. Cook until cranberries pop. Refrigerate overnight. Put cranberries in a crock pot. Add chicken, pepper, and salt. Cover. Set to low. Cook for five hours.

Sticky Chicken

Ingredients

½ tsp black pepper

1 tsp cayenne pepper

½ tsp garlic powder

1 c chopped onion

1 tsp salt

3 to 4 lb roasting chicken

1 tsp onion powder

1 tsp thyme

2 tsp paprika

1 tsp white pepper

Instructions

Put the above spices in small bowl and mix thoroughly. Clean out the chicken. Pat dry. Rub spice mixture on chicken. Don't forget the inside. Put in resealable bag, and let sit in fridge overnight

When ready to bake chicken, let it come to room temp. Heat oven to 275. Place onions in the cavity of the chicken. Place in baking pan. Bake uncovered for five hours. The juices will start to caramelize, and chicken will brown up. Ignore the chicken's pop up thermometer if it has one. When done, take and let it red before you crave it.

Italian Chicken Breasts

Ingredients

Salt

1 c chicken broth

3 c sliced mushrooms

½ tsp pepper blend

4 boneless, skinless chicken breasts

1 tsp Italian seasoning

1 tsp paprika

Instructions

Mix all spices together. Rub this over the chicken. Add chicken to warmed skillet. Cook until browned. Turn and brown another side. Reduce heat. Mix in the broth and mushrooms. Place on lid and let cook for 20 minutes or the chicken reaches 160.

White Chicken Chili

Ingredients

¼ tsp cayenne pepper

2 tsp ground cumin

1 c salsa

2 diced chili peppers

2 seeded, diced jalapenos

1 tbsp olive oil

2 medium chopped onions

1 lb great northern beans (soaked overnight in water)

2 cloves minced garlic

6 cups diced cooked chicken breasts

1 ½ tsp oregano

Instructions

Simmer the beans with half the garlic and onions in chicken broth for two hours. Be sure the beans are soft. Add salsa and chicken.

In olive oil sauté onions, spices, and peppers. Add to bean mixture. Simmer an additional hour.

Serve with reduced fat cheese or light sour cream.

Brown Sugar Garlic Chicken

Ingredients

2 tbsp butter

Black pepper

4 tsp brown sugar

1 clove garlic

12 oz boneless, skinless chicken breast

Instructions

Place butter in a pan and melt. Place in garlic, and cook until it smells. Place in chicken breasts and cook through. Sprinkle with pepper.

When chicken is cooked through, add brown sugar to the top. Allow to melt. This should take about five minutes.

Serve with favorite vegetable. It is great on top of a salad.

Black Bean Soup

Ingredients

2 c chicken broth

1 cup salsa

2 cans black beans, washed and drained

Instructions

Add all ingredients to pot and heat through. Use an immersion blender or put in blender to make it a creamy black bean soup.

Garnish with fresh cilantro or herbs of choice.

Mushrooms and Beef

Ingredients

1 can low-fat cream of mushroom soup

½ cup water

1 lb lean stew meat

8 oz sliced mushrooms

1 packet onion soup mix

Instructions

Brown meat in skillet. Put meat in slow cooker. Place in mushrooms. Mix water, soup mix, and soup. Pour over beef and mushrooms. Cover. Set to low. Cook for eight hours.

Serve over rice or noodles.

Diet Cola Sloppy Joes

Ingredients

2 tbsp white vinegar

1 tbsp Worcestershire sauce

Garlic powder

2 tsp dry mustard

2/3 c reduced sugar ketchup

1 c diet cola

1 lb 96% lean ground beef

Instructions

Brown beef in skillet. Drain. Put beef back in skillet. Place all the rest in and mix well. Cook 15 minutes or until it thickens.

Serve on buns.

Parmesan Tilapia

Ingredients

Pepper

1 tsp garlic powder, divided

4 sprigs fresh dill

¼ c grated parmesan

2 tsp non-fat plain yogurt

2 tsp light mayonnaise

2 tilapia fillets

Instructions

Heat oven to broil.

If filets are frozen, thaw completely. Put cheese, yogurt, and mayonnaise in a bowl. Mix well.

Put aluminum foil on cookie sheet. Spray with cooking spray.

Put tilapia fillets on cookie sheet 2-inches apart. Spread cheese mixture over each filet. Separate dill with hands and sprinkle over fish. Sprinkle with garlic powder and black pepper. Put the cookie sheet in oven about 6 inches below broiler.

Watch this carefully. It will take about five to seven minutes to cook completely. When cheese starts browning, check every 30 seconds. Fish is going to flake easily when cooked fully.

Turn off broiler and leave fish in the oven. Wait five minutes.

Take out of the oven and serve with a favorite side.

Low-fat Cheeseburger Pie

Ingredients

¾ c shredded cheddar cheese

4 tomato slices

1 clove chopped garlic

½ c chopped onion

¾ cup heart smart Bisquick

¼ c water

1 tbsp Worcestershire sauce

1 c fat-free cottage cheese

1 lb ground turkey

1 egg

Instructions

Heat oven to 350.

Brown turkey in skillet. Add garlic and onions.

While cooking, combine water and baking mix until well combined. Roll dough flat to cover pie plate. Place dough in pie plate.

Add Worcestershire to meat.

In additional bowl mix egg and cottage cheese.

Pour turkey mixture into a pie plate. Top with cottage cheese mixture. Top with cheese.

Add on tomatoes. Cook for about 30 to 40 minutes.

Quick Chili

Ingredients

1 tbsp chili powder

½ c salsa

1 tbsp cumin powder

1 15 oz can kidney beans, rinsed and drained

1 28 oz can stewed tomatoes

1 15 oz can pinto beans, rinsed and drained

½ c chopped onion

1 lb ground turkey

Instructions

Brown the turkey with onion. Add salsa, cumin, chili powder, garlic, tomatoes, and beans. Cook until heated through.

Serve with baked potato, cooked rice, cooked pasta, or cornbread. Top with cheese.

Applesauce Peanut Chicken

Ingredients

1 15 oz jar unsweetened applesauce

Salt

Pepper

½ c powdered peanuts

1/8 c Splenda brown sugar

¼ cup yellow mustard

2 ½ lbs chicken pieces

Instructions

Sauté chicken in pan until almost done. Add applesauce, powdered peanuts, brown sugar, and mustard. Stir together. Simmer until chicken temp reaches 165.

Chicken Chili

Ingredients

½ tsp black pepper

3 c water

2 c pinto beans that have soaked overnight in water.

1 tsp salt

1 tbsp chili powder

3 ¼ cups salsa Verde or green enchilada sauce

1 ½ tsp ground cumin

2 cans chopped green chilies

1 ½ c cooked chopped chicken

1 medium chopped onion

Instructions

Sauté chicken and onion with spices until onion is soft. Add beans, water, enchilada sauce, and chilies.

Simmer until beans are tender.

This is good topped with cheese and tortilla chips.

Creamy Chicken

Ingredients

¼ c Italian dressing

1 clove chopped garlic

½ c low sodium chicken broth

1 small chopped onion

1 can low-fat cream of chicken soup

8 oz. low-fat cream cheese

3 lbs boneless, skinless chicken breast

Instructions

Spray slow cooker with nonstick spray.

Put the chicken inside and drizzle with dressing.

Sauté garlic and onions in a pan with cooking spray until soft. Add cream cheese, broth, and soup. Combine until creamy. Add to slow cooker.

Place on lid, set to six hours on low.

Serve with vegetables of choice. Add the vegetables to the crock pot for a one pot meal.

Mexican Chicken Stew

Ingredients

1 can black beans, undrained

1 can chopped green chilies

1 can black olives

1 can Mexican style chili beans, undrained

1 can diced tomatoes

1 pkg taco seasoning

2 to 3 chicken breasts

Instructions

Put chicken in crock pot. Add diced tomatoes, black beans, chili beans, taco seasoning, black olives, chopped green chilies. Don't stir. Cover. Set to low. Cook for eight hours.

Remove the chicken and shred it up. Place it back into the cooker. Mix well. Serve eight on a tortilla or with tortilla chips. Top with shredded cheese, tomatoes, and chopped lettuce.

Stuffed Peppers

Ingredients

1 ½ lbs lean ground beef

1 tsp garlic powder

1 cup chopped onion

1 ½ cups minute rice, brown

1 large egg

1 tsp salt

2 cups tomato sauce

1 tsp black pepper

4 bell peppers

Instructions

Slice all of the peppers in half. Take out the ribs and seeds.

Combine remaining ingredients except for a cup of the tomato sauce and bell peppers.

Split this between the bell peppers

Spread a half cup of the tomato sauce in the slow cooker. Place in the peppers. Top with the rest of the sauce

Place on the lid. Set to low. Cook six hours.

Pork Chops

Ingredients

Salt

Pepper

½ c water

2 tbsp corn starch

1 ½ c chicken broth

2 tbsp olive oil

½ c thin sliced onion

½ c each yellow, red, green bell peppers, sliced thin

4 3 oz pork chops

Instructions

Sauté pork in olive oil until browned. Take out of the pan. Set to the side.

Toss in the pepper and onion in the pan and sauté until they are caramelized and aromatic. Pour in the broth and put the pork back in.

Pork should cook until no longer pink, so about 15 minutes. Remove from pan.

Stir corn starch into cold water until dissolved. Place in the pan and let thicken.

Add pepper and salt to taste.

White Chicken Chili

Ingredients

Parsley flakes
1 red bell pepper, diced and seeded
Onion powder
2 cans low sodium chicken broth
½ diced sweet onion
Garlic powder
Cumin
1 tbsp olive oil
1 to 2 tbsp canned green chilies, drained
1 lb boneless, skinless chicken breast, cubed
1 cup chunky salsa
1 heaping tsp minced garlic

3 cans great northern beans

Instructions

Heat Dutch oven and add olive oil. Mix the onion, garlic, and bell pepper into the pot, and they should cook until soft

Add chicken. Sprinkle with cumin, onion powder, and garlic powder. Brown up until no longer pink

Place in chilies, salsa, chicken broth, and beans. Stir well.

Add ¼ tsp parsley flakes, ½ tsp onion powder, ½ tsp garlic powder, and 1 ½ tsp cumin.

Heat until simmering. Simmer 20 minutes.

If you want it thicker, you can use a slurry of ¼ cup warm water and 3 tbsp corn starch mixed together before adding to pan. Let this simmer a couple more minutes until to desired thickness.

Leftovers freeze extremely well.

Chicken and Artichoke Casserole

Ingredients

1 can reduced-fat cream of mushroom soup

1 14 oz can artichoke hearts, packed in brine, drained

2 lbs. boneless, skinless chicken breast

Instructions

Cut chicken into 2-inch pieces and add to crock pot. Cut artichoke hearts in half. Add to crock pot. Add soup. Cover. Set to low. Cook five hours. Stir to combine. Serve and enjoy.

Baked Chicken and Veggies

Ingredients

Pepper

1 tsp thyme

½ c water

1 chicken, skin removed, cut into pieces

1 quartered large onion

6 sliced carrots

4 sliced potatoes

Instructions

Heat oven to 400. Put onions, carrots, and potatoes in roasting pan. Place chicken on top. Mix pepper, thyme, and water. Pour over vegetables and chicken. Bake at least an hour until tender and browned. Internal temperature should be 165. Baste chicken with juices during cooking.

Black Bean and Pork Verde Stew

Ingredients

1 tsp red pepper flakes

1 14.5 oz can no salt added black beans, washed and drained

2 canned chipotle pepper in adobo sauce, minced

3 garlic cloves

1 tsp ground cumin

1 packet taco seasoning

1 14 oz can no salt added chicken broth

1 ¼ c chopped onions

1 lb pork loin, trimmed and cubed

1 tsp adobo sauce

1 14.5 oz can no salt added diced tomatoes in juice

2 tsp olive oil

Instructions

Heat up a Dutch oven with oil. Place in pork. Cook until browned. Place in garlic and onion cook until softened. Add seasoning packet, cumin, chipotle peppers, and sauce. Stir to mix. Add beans, tomatoes, red pepper flakes, and broth. Stir. Let it come to boil. Let it cook lightly. Cover with a lid and cook for another 40 to 45 minutes or until the pork is tender. Serve in bowls over rice.

Asian Lettuce Wraps

Ingredients

1 small cucumber, seeded and sliced into 1-inch strips
8 small butter lettuce leaves
3 tbsp sherry cooking wine
1 8 oz. can water chestnuts, drained and minced
¼ tsp salt
½ lb ground chicken breast
1 green onion, chopped
1 tsp toasted sesame oil
2 tbsp. hoisin sauce
1 c minced onion
2 packets sugar substitute
1 tbsp unsalted peanut butter
1 tsp minced ginger
2 tsp hot pepper sauce
2 tsp low sodium soy sauce
1 tbsp minced garlic

1 8 oz can bamboo shoots, drained and minced

Instructions

Combine sugar substitute, hot sauce, soy sauce, peanut butter, hoisin sauce, sherry, water chestnuts, and bamboo shoots. Mix well. Set to the side.

Spray skillet with cooking spray. Warm and add in the onion cooking until it turns soft. Stir in garlic, cooking until it smells. Turn up the heat. Add salt, ginger, and ground chicken. Breaking up chicken so that it cooks all the way through. Add bamboo shoot mixture. Heat through. Stir in sesame oil. Take off heat.

Divide chicken equally onto the lettuce leaves. Top with green onion and cucumber. Serve and enjoy.

Black Bean and Turkey Sloppy Joes

Ingredients

1 tsp Mrs. Dash onion and herb blend

1 14.5 oz can diced tomatoes with green chilies

1 ½ c low sodium tomato juice

1 tbsp. olive oil

1 tsp paprika

2 tsp chili powder

1 medium chopped onion

1 tsp minced garlic

1 6 oz can tomato paste

1 14.5 oz can black beans, drained and rinsed

1 lb ground turkey

Instructions

Brown turkey up, and drain the fat off. Place in all of the other ingredients and cook until as thick as you want it.

Serve on buns or bread.

Taco Chicken

Ingredients

¼ c nonfat sour cream

1 c salsa

4 4 oz. chicken breast

1 pkg taco seasoning

Instructions

Heat oven to 375.

Place taco seasoning and chicken in resealable bag. Shake to coat. Place in greased casserole. Bake 30 minutes. Coat the top with salsa five minutes before it's done. Top with sour cream just before serving.

Fajita Chicken

Ingredients

Garlic powder

1 bag frozen pepper and onion blend

3 c chunky salsa

1 packet taco seasoning

3 lb. frozen boneless chicken breast

Instructions

Put frozen chicken breasts in crock pot. Sprinkle with taco seasonings. Spoon some salsa over each one. Sprinkle with garlic powder. Dump frozen peppers and onions on top.

Place on lid and set to eight hours on low.

Serve as is or shred for tacos, fajitas, nachos, taco salad, burritos, or to top a baked potato. You will have leftovers.

Chicken and Vegetables

Ingredients

1 8oz can tomato sauce

3 to 4 cloves minced garlic

3 16 oz cans diced tomatoes

3 lb bag boneless skinless chicken breast

8 oz sliced mushrooms

3 small slice zucchini

4 yellow or red sliced bell peppers

2 small diced Vidalia onions

Instructions

Cube chicken. Place in large pan with garlic and onion. Cook. Season to taste.

Continue to cook unto almost done. Add tomato sauce, canned tomatoes, mushrooms, zucchini, and bell peppers. Place a lid on it and let it cook about 20 minutes. Veggies should be tender.

Serve as is or over rice. Any leftovers freeze well.

Spicy Peanut Vegetarian Chili

Ingredients

1 16 oz can white beans, washed and drained

2 cups vegetable broth

1 c chopped onion

2/3 c powdered peanuts

2 cloves minced garlic

1 28 oz. can diced tomatoes

1 tbsp. peanut oil

1 tsp chipotle chili powder

1 16 oz. can black beans, washed and drained

¼ tsp dried oregano

1 15 oz. can tomato sauce

2 tbsp. chili powder

Instructions

Heat up a Dutch oven with some oil. Place the garlic and onion in and allow them to cook until they turn tender. Stir in salt, oregano, pepper, and chili powder. Cook until fragrant. Add broth, tomato sauce, tomatoes, powdered peanuts, corn, and beans. Let boil. Simmer about 30 minutes.

Halloumi Wraps

Ingredients

Dressing:

1 tsp olive oil

2 tbsp sweet chili sauce

Filing and Salad:

4 wraps, low-carb

6 radishes, sliced

1 lime, juiced

4 spring onions, sliced

2 celery stalks, sliced

1 head lettuce, leaves separated

9 oz. Halloumi cheese

Instructions

Stir all of the dressing parts together.

Slice the halloumi into eight slices and coat them with the dressing.

Place them on a grill or in a pan and brown on both sides for three minutes. They should become brown and crisp on the outside.

While they cook, combine the radishes, spring onions, celery, and lettuce together. Add all the rest of the dressing on your salad and toss everything together.

Split this salad between all of your wraps and place two of the grilled cheese slices on each of them. Serve this immediately.

Sichuan Roasted Eggplant

Ingredients

6 spring onions, chopped – garnish
Drizzle sesame oil – optional
1 tbsp dark soy sauce
3 eggplants
Pepper
2 tbsp olive oil
Salt
2 tsp honey
2 tbsp sweet chili sauce
1 red chili, chopped finely
3 tsp ginger, chopped
2 tbsp tomato paste

4 garlic cloves, crushed

Instructions

You should have your oven at 400. Place foil or a silicone baking sheet onto a cookie sheet, so that clean up is easy.

Combine the pepper, honey, salt, sweet chili sauce, oil, soy sauce, tomato paste, chili, and ginger together.

Slice the eggplants in half lengthwise then make a deep score, crisscross marks into the eggplants. Make sure the skins don't get cut. Put the eggplants on your baking sheet and spoon the paste that you created earlier over all of the halves. Loosely cover eggplants with foil and let them cook for 30 minutes.

Take the foil off of them and let it continue to cook for another 30 minutes. It should be tender and brown. Drizzle the top with some sesame oil if you want to, and let them stand for five minutes.

Top with a scattering of onions.

Vegetable Stir-Fry

Ingredients

Small handful of cilantro – optional

4 tbsp soy sauce

2 red peppers, sliced and cored

11 oz baby corn, halved

2 garlic cloves, crushed

1 lb Chinese leaf lettuce, shredded

1 lb oriental mushrooms

1 onion, sliced

1 chili, chopped finely

2 tsp sesame oil

Instructions

Oil a wok and heat it up over medium heat.

Place the garlic and the chili and let them cook for 30 seconds.

Place in the peppers, corn, Chinese lettuce, and mushrooms. Stir-fry this mixture for about four minutes, or until they become tender-crisp.

Pour the soy sauce over everything and toss it together.

Serve with cilantro.

Lemon Chicken Kebabs

Ingredients

2 tsp basil – garnish

1 tbsp lemon zest

Skewer vegetables – like zucchini and tomatoes

4 chicken breasts, cubed

2 lemons, juice

2 tbsp olive oil

Dipping Sauce:

3 tbsp chopped basil

2 garlic cloves, crushed

8 oz plain goat's cheese yogurt

½ lemon, juice, and zest

Instructions

In a bowl, mix the lemon juice, salt, lemon zest, pepper, and oil. Put the chicken and coat it in the sauce. Place a covering over the bowl and let it marinate in the fridge for around 30 minutes.

While that marinates, combine the pepper, lemon juice, basil, salt, lemon zest, garlic, and yogurt to make the dipping sauce. Place this in the fridge until ready to be used.

Thread the veggies and chicken onto eight to 12 skewers, alternating them. Grill the kebabs for five to eight minutes on every side, making sure to turn them often. Baste them as they cook with the leftover marinade

Once the chicken is done, serve them with the dipping sauce and top with some basil.

Veggie Chilli

Ingredients

Sprigs cilantro – optional garnish

1 tsp chopped rosemary

1 red onion, sliced

½ c strong grated cheese, low-fat

2 tsp chipotle paste

12 oz cherry tomato and basil sauce

14 oz. black beans, washed and drained

7 oz. Romano peppers, sliced and seeded

Nonstick spray, low-fat

Instructions

Coat a skillet with a generous amount of the nonstick spray. Let it heat up and add the rosemary, red onion, and peppers. Let this cook for five minutes.

Place in the chipotle paste, cherry tomato and basil sauce, and beans. Let this mixture simmer for around ten minutes. The peppers should become tender.

Serve the chili with cilantro and grated cheese.

Lamb Koftas

Ingredients

2 tbsp dressing, fat-free
2 tbsp mint, chopped
4 oz feta cheese, light
8 oz cherry tomatoes, halved
½ cucumber, sliced and halved
2 tbsp parsley, chopped
1 ½ oz. craisins
½ tsp ground coriander
½ tsp cumin
1 garlic clove, crushed
½ small onion, chopped
8 oz lean ground lamb

2 oz bulgur wheat

Instructions

Place the wheat into a skillet. Place in water to cover it and let it come up to a boil. Cook five minutes. The wheat should become tender, and drain off the water.

Combine the garlic, onion, wheat, and lamb together. Mix in the parsley, craisins, coriander, and cumin. Mix until everything comes together. Split the meat up into 12 portions.

Heat up your broiler or a grill. Take one of the 12 portions and press around a skewer, tightly, to make an oval. Continue this with the rest of the portions. Put this on a broiler pan or on the grill, and cook for around ten minutes. Make sure you turn them so that they are cooked through and browned on both sides.

Meanwhile, combine the rest of the parsley, mint, feta, tomatoes, and cucumbers and toss them in the dressing. Serve with the koftas.

Beef and Broccoli Stir-Fry

Ingredients

4 scallions, shredded

1 tsp rice vinegar

4 tbsp oyster sauce

2 red chilies, sliced thinly

5 oz shiitake mushrooms, sliced

8 oz broccoli, cut in half

1 red onion, sliced thickly

Low-fat spray

12 oz beef steak, cut into ½ inch strips

1 tsp ginger, grated

1 tbsp light soy sauce

Instructions

Combine the steak, ginger, and soy sauce and allow the steak to sit for 15 minutes.

Spray a wok with low-fat spray. Let it heat up and place in the steak mixture. For four to five minutes, stir-fry the steak until browned and cooked. Place the steak in a clean bowl for later.

Place the chili, mushrooms, broccoli, and onion in the wok and let it cook for five minutes, or until all the veggies have become tender. Add a little water or more low-fat spray when needed to make sure that it doesn't burn.

Place the steak and its juices back to the wok and mix in the rice vinegar and oyster sauce. Cook for another couple of minutes until everything is good and heated through.

Garnish with a scattering of scallions.

Thai Sea Bass

Ingredients

1 tbsp soy sauce

2 tbsp chopped cilantro – optional

2 sea bass fillets

2 garlic cloves, crushed

3 tbsp. oil

4 tsp ginger, grated

1 lemon, juice and zest

1 mild red chili, sliced and seeded

2 spring onions, chopped

8 oz. bok choy, quartered

1 tbsp. fish sauce

4 oz. asparagus, trimmed

Instructions

Your oven should be at 400.

Put the onions, bok choy, and asparagus into a roasting pan.

Mix together the lemon juice, lemon zest, fish sauce, oil, ginger, soy sauce, chili, and garlic together. Pour the mixture over the vegetables and toss to coat. Then, place the veggies in the oven and allow it to cook for five minutes.

Take them out and set the sea bass on top. Place this for another eight minutes in the oven, or until your sea bass is cooked all the way through. It should flake easily with poked with a fork, and it should be opaque.

Place the rest of the dressing over the fish, top with cilantro, and enjoy.

Mini Meatloaves

Ingredients

Toppings: dill pickle, mustard, or ketchup – these are optional

¾ c shredded cheese, reduced-fat

¼ tsp pepper

1 tsp onion powder

1 lb. ground beef, extra lean

2 tsp mustard

1 c onion, chopped

½ tsp salt

1 tsp garlic powder

3 tbsp. ketchup

¼ c egg whites

¼ c panko breadcrumbs, whole wheat

½ c green bell pepper, chopped

Instructions

Your oven should be set at 375. Coat a regular cupcake tin with cooking spray.

Mix together all of the above, except for the cheese. Make sure it is well combined. Distribute the meat into between the cup and smooth across the tops.

Bake them for 35 minutes or until the edges have browned up and it is firm.

Grate some cheese and sprinkle it on top and return it to the oven for another three minutes to melt the cheese.

Serve with the desired toppings.

Stuffed Chicken

Ingredients

Pepper

Salt

Tomato sauce

Mozzarella cheese

½ c ricotta cheese

½ pack of frozen spinach, squeezed

1 egg

¼ c parmesan, divided

½ c breadcrumbs

4 chicken cutlets, pounded thin

Instructions

Combine half of the parmesan with the breadcrumbs and place on the side.

Mix the remaining parmesan, spinach, and ricotta together in a bowl. You should make sure that the spinach has been completely squeezed dry.

Place the cutlets onto a cutting board spread two tablespoons of the spinach mixture over the top.

Roll the cutlets up and secure with toothpicks.

In a shallow dish beat up the eggs.

Coat cutlets in egg and then the breadcrumbs.

Put the cutlets seam side down into a casserole dish that is coated with nonstick spray. Your oven should be at 425. Bake 25 minutes.

Take the casserole dish out and top with tomato sauce and mozzarella.

Cook for another five minutes and enjoy.

Chicken Nuggets

Ingredients

Nonstick spray

2 tbsp parmesan

3 tbsp. panko breadcrumbs

¼ tsp pepper

¼ tsp oregano

½ tsp garlic salt

½ tsp Italian herbs

½ tsp salt

3 tsp canola oil

1 lb chicken breasts, diced

Instructions

Your oven should be at 450.

Toss the chicken with the oil. Sprinkle with the pepper, oregano, garlic salt, Italian herbs, and salt. Massage all of the spices into you chicken.

Place the parmesan cheese, panko, and the chicken into a bag and seal the bag closed. Shake the bag and squeeze the chicken a few times to get it coated well.

Grease up a cookie sheet with baking spray.

Place the chicken nuggets on the cookie sheet in one layer.

Spritz the top of the chicken with more baking spray.

Cook it for about eight minutes or until t

Let it cook for eight minutes, or until it is no longer pink.

Crustless Pizza Bites

Ingredients

Pizza toppings of your choice

Pizza sauce

Mozzarella cheese, shredded

Thick cut Canadian bacon

Instructions

First, you need to grease up your regular muffin tin. Place three Canadian bacon slices like a three leaf clover over the cups. Press down gently to press them into the cups. They don't like to stay that will, but it will be okay. Once you add the toppings, it will settle better.

Gather together your cheese, sauce, and toppings.

Place a tablespoon of the pizza sauce into each of the pizza cups.

Add in as many pizza toppings as you want, and as your cups can hold.

Sprinkle over with a good amount of the mozzarella cheese.

Your oven should be at 350. Place the pizza inside and bake it for 27 minutes or until things start to golden and it becomes bubbly. Make sure not to burn the pizza.

Pop the pizzas out with a fork. A small amount of juice may be in the bottom of the cup, just discard that. Enjoy the pizzas either with a fork or by hand.

Mini Chicken Parmesan

Ingredients

¾ c mozzarella cheese, reduced-fat
¾ c pasta sauce
2 cloves garlic, minced
¾ c parmesan cheese
1/3 tsp pepper
¾ tsp dried thyme
¾ tsp salt
½ small onion, chopped
¾ tsp oregano
¾ tsp dried basil
6 tbsp breadcrumbs
1 egg white
1 egg

1 ½ lb ground chicken breast

Instructions

Your oven should be at 350. Lightly coat a regular muffin tin with some non-stick spray.

Mix together the parmesan, pepper, onion, salt, garlic, oregano, thyme, basil, breadcrumbs, egg whites, egg, and chicken. Do not overmix. Fold the mixture just until you see everything is well incorporated and is distributed throughout the chicken.

Place the mixture evenly between the 12 cups. Place the pasta sauce over the muffins. Place this in your oven and cook 20 minutes. Take it out of the oven and add around a tablespoon of shredded cheese and place it back in the oven for another two minutes making sure the cheese melt on top. Pop them out with a knife or fork and enjoy.

Desserts

Coconut Pistachio Fingers

Ingredients

Extra pistachios

¼ c coconut flakes, unsweetened

2 tbsp olive oil

4 tbsp sugar-free syrup – or maple or agave syrup

Pinch salt

1 c rolled oats

1 c shelled pistachio

Instructions

Your oven should be set at 350. Place greased foil or parchment paper in an eight-inch square dish.

Put the salt, pistachios, and oats in your food processor and pulse them up until they are very fine.

Turn on the processor, and while it's running, add in the oil and syrup until it starts to form a crumbly but moist dough. It shouldn't stick together yet.

Place this in the dish and press it down with a spoon until level. Sprinkle the extra pistachios and the coconut flakes on top.

Bake this for 12 minutes. It should be cooked through and golden. Lift the cookies out by lifting up the foil or parchment. Let it cool on a rack.

Cut it into 16 long cookies and keep it stored in a container.

Peanut Butter Muffins

Ingredients

4 tbsp protein powder

½ c mini chocolate chips

½ tsp salt

1 tbsp vanilla

¼ c honey

2 eggs

1 c creamy peanut

1 tsp baking powder

2 bananas, extremely ripe

Instructions

Your oven should be at 400.

Place the above, except chocolate chips, into your blender. Mix everything up for around 30 seconds, or until it is well mixed.

Place in a bowl and lightly mix in the chocolate chips.

Spray a regular muffin tin with nonstick spray and add batter into each cup.

Cook these for 12 to 14 minutes, or until they have set.

PB Mug Cake

Ingredients

1 tbsp chopped peanuts

1/8 tsp vanilla

1 tbsp powdered peanut butter

1 tbsp vanilla soymilk, light

2 tbsp egg whites

½ packet of sweetener

¼ tsp baking powder

1 tbsp vanilla protein powder

1 tbsp coconut flour

Instructions

Coat a mug with cooking spray. Place in the sweetener, baking powder, powdered peanut butter, protein powder, and flour. Combine everything together.

Mix in two tablespoons of water, vanilla extract, soymilk, and egg whites.

Place in the microwave for a minute and 15 seconds, or until it has set up.

Slide a knife around the cake. Set a plate over the cup and quickly flip it. Shake the cake free from the cup. Top with some extra peanuts.

Salted Caramel Cheesecakes

Ingredients

Crust:
2/3 c lightly sweetened fiber cereal
2 tbsp Greek yogurt cream cheese, low-fat and softened
Filling:
½ c sweetener
1/3 c whey protein powder, unflavored
4 oz salted caramel Greek yogurt, fat-free
1 egg

8 oz Greek yogurt cream cheese, low-fat and softened

Instructions

Crust:

Your oven should be at 325.

Place parchment into the bottom of four mini spring form pans.

Pulse up the cream cheese and the cereal until it becomes clumpy. Press the crust into each of the pans and bake them for about ten minutes.

Cheesecake:

Beat together the sweetener, protein powder, vanilla, yogurt, egg, and cream cheese. Beat at medium speed for a minute and then increase it to high for another two minutes. Make sure all of the lumps have been removed.

Place the cream cheese over the crust. Put the pans into a casserole dish. Put boiling water into a separate baking dish a sit it on the bottom rack of your oven. Put the dish of cheesecakes on the middle rack. Let this bake for 30 minutes.

Switch your oven off and slightly crack your oven door. Let them stay there until the cool.

Carefully release the spring form pan and slide the cheesecake off by the parchment paper.

Mini Strawberry Cheesecakes

Ingredients

Crust:

1 tbsp sugar

¼ c butter, melted

1 c graham cracker crumbs

Filling:

5 drops red food coloring

2 5oz containers Greek yogurt, strawberry

2 eggs

¼ tsp salt

½ c strawberry jams

2/3 c sugar

1 tbsp cornstarch

1 tsp vanilla

2 8oz pack 1/3 fat cream cheese

Topping:

15 strawberries

1 c whipped cream, fat-free

Instructions

Crust:

Your oven should be at 325. Put liners into a regular muffin tin.

Mix together the sugar, butter, and graham crackers. Press a tablespoon of this into every one of the cupcakes tins

Filling:

Beat together the sugar, salt, cornstarch, and creams cheese until it becomes fluffy. Mix in the food coloring, vanilla, and strawberry jam. Make sure it is mixed well. Mix an egg one at a time. Stir in the Greek yogurt.

Pour the mixture into the cups over the crusts. The liners should be filled almost all the way to the top. Cook for 20 to 22 minutes. The edges should be set with the centers wobbly

Let them cool for 30 minutes. Set them out on a wire rack and allow them to completely cool. Place in the fridge for at least four hours before you serve them.

Top the cheese cake with whipped cream and strawberries.

Blueberry Cookies

Ingredients

2 scoops vanilla protein powder

1 c berries

½ c oatmeal

4 egg whites

Instructions

Stir the oatmeal, egg whites, and protein powder together until well combined.

Mix in the berries of your choice.

Drop spoonfuls of you cookie dough onto a nonstick coated cookie sheet.

Your oven should be at 425. Bake them for 10 to 15 minutes.

Strawberry Cheesecake

Ingredients

4 tsp Splenda

2 c strawberries, halved

½ fat-free cool whip

1 c nonfat milk

½ pkg sugar-free cheesecake pudding

4 oz. fat-free ricotta cheese

Instructions

Wash strawberries and cut them in half. Add Splenda and gently mix. Set to the side.

Add milk, pudding mix, and ricotta to blender. Blend until creamy and smooth. Pour into a bowl but not with the strawberries. Add cool whip and gently fold.

Spoon a small amount of the pudding mix into serving dishes. Add strawberries. Continue layering there you have used up all ingredients. Top with any remaining strawberries.

Pumpkin Pie Cheesecake

Ingredients

¼ tsp ground allspice

4 egg whites

½ tsp ground cinnamon

1 c canned pumpkin

¼ tsp ground nutmeg

1 c sugar substitute

3 8 oz. pkg fat-free cream cheese

1 tsp vanilla extract

Instructions

Heat oven to 375.

Blend vanilla, sugar, and cream cheese together in a bowl with electric mixer. Add spices, eggs, and pumpkin. Blend until it is smooth.

Pour into a 9-inch spring form pan. You can use a pie crust if wanted.

Bake between 60 and 70 minutes until top turns lightly brown. Remove and cool to room temp

Refrigerate until it is chilled.

Once chilled, remove from spring form pan and cut.

Serve with the fat-free cool whip or whipped cream.

Apple Cake

Ingredients

¼ c chopped walnuts

1 tsp cinnamon

1 c all-purpose flour

½ tsp salt

½ tsp baking powder

4 tbsp butter

4 medium diced apples

½ tsp baking soda

½ tsp nutmeg

1 c Splenda

1 egg

Instructions

Heat oven to 350.

Peel, core, and dice the apples.

Grease an 8-inch square pan.

Blend butter and sugar together.

Beat egg, add walnuts and vanilla. Combine. Add to apples. Add butter mixture and mix it together.

Sift remaining ingredients and add to apple mixture. Mix well. Pour into prepared pan. Cook about 45 minutes. Allow it to cool and then cut into squares.

Fruit Dip

Ingredients

6 oz. fat-free, sugar-free vanilla yogurt

8 oz. low-fat cream cheese, softened

3 tbsp. Splenda

1 tsp vanilla

Instructions

Beat up the cream cheese. Add Splenda, vanilla, and yogurt slowly. Increase speed and blend until fluffy and light.

Use as a dip for favorite fruit.

Mousse

Ingredients

2 c boiling water

3 scoops vanilla protein powder

2 small boxes sugar free jello favorite flavor

24 oz 1% cottage cheese

Instructions

Boil two cups water. Add jello and stir until dissolved. Let cool a few minutes.

But cottage cheese into a blender. Blend out the lumps.

Mix in cooled jello and protein powder. Blend until well mixed.

Divide into six serving dishes. Chill overnight. This will have a very light mousse-like consistency.

Serve and enjoy.

Cheesecake Pudding

Ingredients

1 cup plain fat-free Greek yogurt

1 pkg sugar-free cheesecake pudding mix

Instructions

Mix all of the above ingredients together.

I Can't Believe It's Not Cheesecake

Ingredients

1 small pkg sugar-free flavored gelatin, your choice of flavor

2 tbsp. Splenda

2 8 oz. pkg low-fat cream cheese

1 cup boiling water

1 6 oz container Greek yogurt, plain

Instructions

Mix water and gelatin until dissolved. Add cream cheese and yogurt. Mix with electric mixer until thoroughly combined. Taste. Add Splenda if needed.

Put in fridge overnight.

Once ready to serve, garnish with fruit, sugar-free cookie crumbs, or whipped cream.

Strawberry Dessert

Ingredients

4 c fresh sliced strawberries

2 8 oz tubs light cool whip

2 small boxes sugar-free strawberry jello

32 oz container 4% cottage cheese

Instructions

Combine jello mix and cottage cheese. Combine. Mix in the cool whip and strawberries. Chill.

Pumpkin Protein Pie

Ingredients

2 scoops unflavored whey protein

2 oz. pkg pecan halves

1 tsp nutmeg

½ tsp salt

1/3 cup Splenda

1 tsp cinnamon

1 c ricotta cheese, low-fat

1 c nonfat milk

2 large eggs

2 c pumpkin puree

Instructions

Heat oven to 350. Spray 4 small ramekins and 9-inch pie plate with cooking spray.

Blend ½ cup milk, eggs, and ricotta cheese until smooth. It will be liquid.

Add all the rest and mix up again.

Place into sprayed cooking dishes. Place pecans on top.

Bake 45 minutes or until middle is almost solid. There should be no jiggle if cooked through. The center and sides will brown and grow to double the size. If yours starts to burn, reduce temperature to 325 for rest of cooking time.

Take it out from the oven and allow it to cool for one hour before you cut. Slice it into 12 equal pieces. Wipe between cuts.

Silky Chocolate Dessert

Ingredients

¼ tsp peppermint extract

1 pkg sugar-free chocolate fudge instant pudding

1 tbsp cocoa powder

½ tsp vanilla extract

16 oz silken tofu

1 c skim milk

¼ c hot water

1 envelope unflavored gelatin

Instructions

Mix unflavored gelatin and hot water in small bowl. Set aside and let firm.

Combine instant pudding mix and milk in another bowl. Dice tofu into cubes and put in a bowl alongside of the pudding. Whisk vigorously to break up soy cubes. Add peppermint extract, cocoa powder, and vanilla.

Spoon into a blender. Blend smooth. You might have to shake the blender, so ingredients don't stick. When the mixture has reached a smoothie consistency, add gelatin until combined. Blend one more time.

Pour into 8-inch glass pie plate. Cover and put in the fridge for about 30 minutes to get firm. Cut into eight equal pieces and enjoy.

Snacks and Appetizers

Potato and Crab Salad

Ingredients

Lemon wedge

Smoked salmon and green salad – optional

Pepper

Salt

4 tbsp snipped chives

½ lemon, juiced

2 tbsp Greek yogurt, fat-free

2 tbsp mayonnaise, extra light

6 oz cooked crab meat

8 medium potatoes, cooked

Instructions

Dice up the potatoes up and put them in a bowl with your flaked crab meat.

Mix together the pepper, chives, salt, lemon juice, yogurt, and mayonnaise. Adjust the pepper and salt as you need to.

Place the mixed dressing over the crab and potatoes and toss together, so it's all well coated.

Serve this with some smoked salmon and a green salad along with a lemon wedge for a complete meal.

Blackberry and Chicken Salad

Ingredients

2 sprigs thyme, chopped

½ to 1 tsp honey

½ lemon, zest

2 tbsp vinaigrette dressing, fat-free or low-fat

1 c blackberries

2 oz feta cheese, light

1 bunch watercress, trimmed

1 cooked chicken breast, shredded

2 tsp olive oil

2 slices walnut bread, chunked

Instructions

Your oven should be at 400. Place the bread onto a cookie sheet and top with oil. Bake these for about five minutes or until the crisp up.

Put the blackberries, feta, watercress, and chicken in a bowl. Top with the fresh croutons.

Combine the thyme, honey, lemon, and vinaigrette and stir well. Place the mixture on top of the salad and toss everything together.

Caprese Salad

Ingredients

Pepper

Salt

2 to 3 tbsp balsamic dressing

Handful salad leaves

7 oz mozzarella, light and sliced

1 ripe avocado, scoop into balls – dip them in lemon juice to keep from oxidizing

6 oz strawberries, sliced

Instructions

Mix together the salad leaves, mozzarella, avocado, and strawberries

Drizzle the balsamic dressing over the top and add a generous amount of pepper and salt.

Toss everything together and enjoy.

Grape Salad

Ingredients

½ c chopped walnuts or pecans

¼ c brown sugar

4 tsp vanilla extract

½ c Splenda

8 oz. fat-free sour cream

2 to 4 lbs red or green grapes

Instructions

Wash and dry grapes. Put grapes in large bowl. Using a hand mixer, blend vanilla, Splenda, sour cream, and cream cheese until mixed well.

Fold into grapes until well coated. Put in 9 X 13 cake pan. Top with the brown sugar and chopped nuts.

Put in refrigerator for an hour.

Chicken Salad

Ingredients

3 tbsp miracle whip light

½ c quartered grapes

¼ c craisins

¼ c diced celery

1 ½ c diced, grilled chicken breast

Instructions

Place all ingredients in a bowl. May be served over a bed of greens or as a sandwich.

Corn and Black Bean Salad

Ingredients

¼ tsp black pepper

1 tsp honey

2 tbsp olive oil

1 tsp lemon juice

¼ c balsamic vinegar

Salt

2 cans 16 oz black beans, drained and rinsed

2 tbsp minced red onion

¼ c chopped fresh parsley

1 tsp minced garlic

1 c whole kernel corn

Instructions

Mix parsley, onion, black beans, and corn together in large bowl.

Whisk pepper, salt, honey, garlic, lemon juice, olive oil, balsamic vinegar together.

Pour over corn and black beans. Stir to coat.

Let stand for 30 minutes.

Serve over a bed of lettuce, with pita chips, or tortilla chips.

Aunt Faye's Chicken Salad

Ingredients

¼ c sliced almonds

1 c red seedless grapes, halved

1 c light sour cream

¼ c light miracle whip

½ tsp celery seed

3 tbsp lemon juice

3 lb cooked, cubed chicken breast

Instructions

Put chicken in large bowl. Add lemon juice, celery seed, sour cream, miracle whip. Stir well. Add almonds and grapes. Give another stir. Place in refrigerator for one hour.

Serve with crackers or flour tortillas.

Grape and Chicken Salad

Ingredients

¼ c walnuts

2 tbsp light mayonnaise

1 c sliced grapes

1 lb grilled chicken

Instructions

Mix everything up in a bowl. Place on a sandwich or lettuce bed.

Baked Zucchini

Ingredients

1 oz 1% milk

1 large egg white

½ c Italian bread crumbs

2 tbsp grated parmesan

2 c sliced zucchini

Instructions

Your oven should be at 400. Spray the baking sheet with nonstick spray.

Combine the dry ingredients in shallow dish.

Stir the milk and egg whites together in a different shallow dish.

Place zucchini slices in milk mixture. Cover with bread crumbs.

Lay in one layer on baking sheet. Spritz with oil spray.

Fry for ten minutes and then flip them over. Fry for another ten minutes until it has crisped up and browned

Salmon Cakes

Ingredients

Salt

1 tsp garlic powder

1 large egg

1 tsp pepper

1 can salmon

1 c diced onion

Instructions

Check salmon for bones and remove. This step gets messy.

Combine everything and make them into patty shapes. Fry like you would a hamburger.

Serve like a hamburger or over a bed of greens.

Standard Chicken Salad

Ingredients

Salt
Pepper
Pinch cayenne
Pinch curry powder
1 tsp mustard
3 tbsp light mayonnaise
1 ½ c chopped celery

1 ½ c cooked, chopped chicken

Instructions

Mix all ingredients well. Season to taste. Place on a lettuce bed.

Deviled Eggs

Ingredients

1 tsp pepper
2 cloves crushed garlic
1 tsp salt
1 tsp onion powder
3 tbsp. fat-free mayonnaise
3 tbsp. Dijon mustard
6 hard-boiled eggs

Instructions

Slice in half long way. Gently take out the yolks and place in a bowl. Use a fork and mash the yolks until fine. Add remaining ingredients. Mix well. Using spoon, place yolk mixture into egg whites.

Hummus

Ingredients

¼ tsp salt

1 tsp chopped garlic

¾ c plain nonfat yogurt

1 16 oz can chickpeas or garbanzo beans

1 ½ tbsp. lemon juice

Instructions

Drain and rinse beans. Put this stuff in your food processor. Mix up until creamy and smooth

Taste test and adjust seasoning if needed. Add cilantro, red pepper, and cumin if desired.

Serve with pita chips or tortilla chips.

Cucumber Soup

Ingredients

1 medium seeded and diced tomato
Salt
Pepper
3 tbsp chopped dill
1 scallion chopped include green parts
1 English cucumber, chunked
2 tsp olive oil
3 cups plain nonfat yogurt

Instructions

Combine dill, scallion, cucumber, and yogurt in a blender. Pulse until smooth. Taste and season accordingly. Ladle into bowls. Top with diced tomato, a drizzle of olive oil and dill sprig.

Serve with a piece of whole grain bread.

Tuna Patties

Ingredients

1 tbsp parmesan cheese
Dash garlic powder
1 large egg
Dash onion powder
1 tbsp light mayonnaise
2 tbsp flax meal
1 pouch tuna in water

Instructions

Drain tuna. Mash with a fork to make smaller. Mix all ingredients with a fork. Form into four patties. Fry in sauté pan greased with nonstick spray until it has browned.

Black Bean Salad

Ingredients

3 cloves garlic, minced

1 tbsp diced cilantro

1 onion, chopped

1 tsp cumin

1 can whole kernel corn, drained

¼ cup apple cider vinegar

1 tsp cayenne pepper

1 tbsp olive oil

1 red bell pepper, chopped and seed removed

¼ cup water

1 can black beans, washed and drained

Instructions

Sauté the onion and the bell pepper together in the oil until they become soft. Mix in garlic, cook until it smells. Add cayenne, cumin, cilantro, corn, vinegar, water, and black beans. Let it come to a boil. Turn it to simmer. When the mixture has reduced slightly, it is ready to eat.

Serve with pita or tortilla chips.

Tuna and Apple Sandwich

Ingredients

3 lettuce leaves

6 slices whole wheat bread

½ tsp honey

1 tsp mustard

¼ c low-fat vanilla yogurt

1 apple

1 can tuna, packed in water, drained

Instructions

Wash the apple. Peel, core, and chop. Put the apple in a bowl. Add tuna, honey, mustard, and yogurt. Stir well. Spread ½ cup onto three slices of bread. Top with lettuce leaves and the other slice of bread.

Chicken Cheesesteak Wrap

Ingredients

2 tsp sliced pickled hot chili peppers

1 whole wheat flour tortilla

¼ lb boneless skinless chicken breast

1 wedge swiss cheese spread

½ c sliced mushrooms

¼ c sliced green pepper

¼ c chopped onion

Instructions

Put chicken on cutting board and pound to ¼-inch thickness. Slice into strips. Spray the skillet with a nonstick cooking spray, or you can brush it with a very little amount of oil as an alternative.

Place the onion and the chicken cooking until the chicken is done. Mix in mushrooms and green peppers. Cook until mushrooms and pepper are soft.

Put tortilla between two damp paper towels. Microwave 20 seconds.

Put tortilla on a plate and put Swiss cheese in a strip down the middle. Top with mushrooms, onions, peppers, and chicken. Add pickled chili peppers. Fold sides over the middle. Serve and enjoy.

Faux Fried Rice

Ingredients

Olive oil spray
2 large egg whites
1 tsp chili paste
¼ c frozen peas
¾ c cooked brown rice
1 clove minced garlic
1 tsp mustard
¼ c chopped carrot
½ c finely chopped green onions
2 tbsp low sodium soy sauce
Pepper
3 oz boneless, skinless chicken breast, cubed
1 tsp toasted sesame oil

Instructions

Combine sesame oil, chili paste, mustard, and soy sauce in small bowl. Set to the side for later use.

Place pepper on chicken. Coat a pan with nonstick spray. Once heated, place chicken in skillet.

Cook all the way through so that it is no longer pink.

Keep the chicken warm.

Spray skillet again with nonstick spray. Add garlic, carrot, and green onions. Cook a few minutes. Add peas and rice. Cook for two minutes so that everything is heated.

Create a hole in the center of rice. Lightly spray exposed part with cooking spray. Add egg whites. Stir to mix into rice. Cook until egg is cooked through.

Put chicken back into the pan. Stir well. Add soy sauce mixture. Continue to cook constantly stirring until heated.

Serve and enjoy.

Ranch Style Salad

Ingredients

2 tbsp garlic and herb soft cheese, light

4 oz bag baby leaf herb salad

1 romaine lettuce head, torn roughly

3 tbsp white wine vinegar

¾ c hard cheese, grated and low-fat

1 red pepper, chopped and seeded

14 oz. kidney beans, washed and drained

11 oz sweet corn

Low-fat spray

Instructions

Spray a generous amount of low-fat spray on your skillet and let it heat up. Add in the sweet corn and let it cook until charred a little.

Combine the cheese, red pepper, and kidney beans together. Stir in the salad leaves and the lettuce.

For the dressing combine three tablespoons of water, the vinegar, and the soft cheese. Add the corn and then drizzle on the dressing. Toss everything together.

Zucchini Chips

Ingredients

Salt

Pepper

1 tbsp parsley, chopped

3 tbsp parmesan, grated

Nonstick spray

3 zucchini, sliced into chips

Instructions

Your oven should be at 425. Place parchment paper onto a rimmed cookie sheet. Put the zucchini slices on the cookie sheet and spray them with some non-stick spray. Combine the salt, parsley, pepper, and parmesan together. Sprinkle this over the zucchini chips. Bake this until the cheese melts, and the zucchini has crisped up but hasn't burned. This should take about 30 minutes.

Mozzarella Sticks

Ingredients

1 tsp olive oil

½ c marinara sauce – dipping

8 wonton wrappers

4 string cheese sticks, halved

1 egg

Instructions

In a bowl, mix together a tablespoon of water and the egg. One at a time, brush each of the wrappers with the egg wash.

Put a string cheese half in the middle of each one of the wrappers; there should be a corner at each end and top and bottom of the wrapper. Take the bottom corner and fold it over the cheese. Bring the two side corners in, and then roll the cheese stick up to the top corner. Make sure you are careful and don't tear the wrappers.

Add some of the olive oil into your skillet and let heat. Place the mozzarella sticks and cook them until they are golden.

Serve with the marinara sauce.

Ranch Cauliflower Bites

Ingredients

1 tsp chives

6 bacon strips, cooked and crumbled

1 ¼ cheddar cheese, shredded and divided

1 ranch seasoning packet

2 egg

1 cauliflower head

Instructions

Your oven should be at 375.

Place the cauliflower in your food processor and pulse it up until it becomes large crumbs.

Put the cauliflower crumbs on a cheesecloth or paper towels and wring out any excess water. Place the drained cauliflower into a bowl.

Add in the chives, ¾ s of the bacon, ranch seasoning, one cup of cheese, and the eggs.

Spray a regular muffin tin with nonstick spray and then fill them up to 2/3s full. Sprinkle the top with bacon and cheese. Place them in the oven for around 20 to 22 minutes. They will turn golden. Top with additional chives if desired.

Peanut Butter Roll-Up

Ingredients

½ tbsp honey

½ banana

1 tbsp peanut butter

1 flatbread

Instructions

Spread your peanut butter over you flatbread. Slice up the banana and place them over the flatbread on top of the peanut butter. Drizzle the honey over everything. Roll it up, slice in half, and then enjoy.

Extras

Blueberry and Basil Water

Ingredients

1-pint blueberries

Bunch of basil

Pitcher of water

Instructions

Rinse blueberries and basil. Crush blueberries and place in the water pitcher. Leave basil on stems and add to pitcher. Fill with water. Refrigerate for a few hours. When you let it sit for a while, it will taste better. You can just keep adding water to the fruit.

Mint and Cucumber Water

Ingredients

3 English cucumber

1 bunch mint

Pitcher of water

Instructions

Rinse cucumber and mint. Thinly slice the cucumbers and place in pitcher. The more cucumbers, the more the water will be flavored. Leave mint on stems add to pitcher. Fill with water. Refrigerate for a few hours. The longer it sits, the better the flavor. You can keep adding water to the pitcher for more flavored water.

Watermelon Water

Ingredients

1 small watermelon

Pitcher of water

Instructions

Cube watermelon and put in pitcher. The more watermelon, the faster the water will be flavored. You may add mint if you prefer. Let sit for several hours. If you let it sit for a while, it will taste better. You can reuse the fruit by adding more water to the pitcher.

Sugar-free Lemonade with Strawberries

Ingredients

1-quart strawberries

1 lemon thinly sliced

Pitcher of water

Instructions

Rinse strawberries. Grate strawberries into a pitcher. Add lemons. Let sit several hours in the refrigerator. The longer it sits, the better the taste. The fruit can be reused by adding more water.

Infused Ice Cubes

Ingredients

Ice cube tray

Boiling water

Herbs and fruits of choice

Instructions

Add any chopped fruit or herbs to ice cube tray. Pour boiling water over. Let cool before you place it in the freezer. When you heat the fruits and herbs, you release their flavor. This gives the ice cube flavor.

Peanut Salad Dressing

Ingredients

1/8 tsp garlic powder

1 tbsp. water

1 tsp Splenda brown sugar

¼ tsp Szechuan chili sauce

1 tbsp. low sodium soy sauce

¼ tsp ground pepper

1/8 tsp sesame oil

2 tbsp. powdered peanuts

Instructions

Put the above in a blender and mix well. Refrigerate any leftovers.

Conclusion

Thank for making it through to the end of *Gastric Bypass Cookbook*. Let's hope it was informative and able to provide you with all of the tools you need to achieve your goals.

The next step is to use these books to make sure that you have success after your gastric bypass surgery.

Finally, if you found this book useful in any way, a review on Amazon is always appreciated!

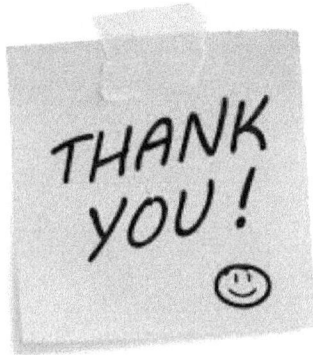

Gastric Bypass Diet

Step By Step Guide
to Gastric Bypass Surgery

Bonus:
FREE Report Reveals The Secrets To Lose Weight

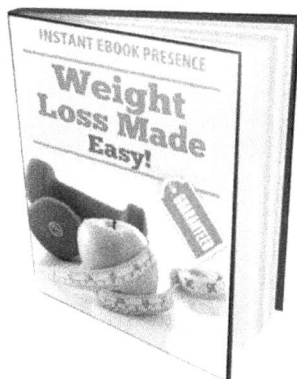

Weight loss doesn't happen from dieting only. Diets are short term solutions to shed extra weight. Diets do not work in the long term because people hate being on a diet (it's ok, you can admit that here). The only long term solution for permanent weight loss is to create new eating habits. This doesn't mean that chocolate will never pass your lips again, but it does mean looking after yourself and watching what you eat...

You can lose weight when you have the right reasons and motivation, and a part of this guide is to help you to find the motivation you need to change your weight...

Go to Get This Guid For FREE

http://www.sportsforsoul.com/weight-loss-2/

Table of Contents

Introduction

Congratulations on downloading your personal copy of *Gastric Bypass Diet Guide.* Thank you for doing so.

The following chapters will discuss some of the many aspects of the gastric bypass surgery.

You will discover how important researching everything about gastric bypass surgery is. This book tells you what gastric bypass is. It will help you decide if this surgery is right for you. It will help tell you what to expect before the surgery. It will teach you what you can and can't eat after your surgery. There are tips for when you are hitting a rough spot.

The final chapter will explore the types of exercises you can do to get your body into the best shape of its life.

There are plenty of books on this subject on the market, thanks again for choosing this one! Every effort was made to ensure it is full of as much useful information as possible. Please enjoy!

What is Gastric Bypass?

Surgery for weight loss was created using different approaches. One approach uses restriction techniques that will limit the number of calories you are able to have. The other focuses on malabsorption. This restricts the calories that the body absorbs.

The first attempted procedure was the juju no-ileal bypass that was performed by A.J. Kremen. He did this procedure in 1954. It centered around the last technique. This procedure was not very good because it caused nutritional deficiencies. The bypassed section of the intestines was too much.

Due to the attempted procedures, there were many different combinations of the procedures developed including Gastric Bypass, Biliopancreatic Diversion, and Duodenal Switch.

These procedures don't try malabsorption. These procedures only use restriction. This creates a smaller stomach that is still usable. Surgeons can bypass a tiny portion of the patient's intestines by incorporating both restriction and malabsorption. This reduces nutritional deficiencies. The smaller stomach limits how much a person can eat.

Mason and Ito performed the first Gastric Bypass procedure in 1967. The procedure has been changed through the years into the form we know today.

This procedure is called Roux-En-Y Gastric Bypass. This surgery can be done two different ways: the laparoscopic and open procedure. The laparoscopic procedure uses five small incisions to lower pain after the operation and to speed up recovery. Meaning you won't have to stay in the hospital as long.

The laparoscopic procedure has been done a lot. Each case was studied. The benefits and hazards were evaluated. Most of the time it is covered by insurance.

It is a great solution to help with weight loss and needs to be considered by anyone who thinks this surgery if for them.

The most popular surgery has been the gastric bypass. The gastric sleeve procedure has become popular since 2011. It was the most popular option in 2015. This doesn't take anything away from how good gastric bypass is. The most reliable procedure is still considered to be gastric bypass. Here is why:

- Long term success with weight loss. Studies reveal that 90 percent of patients keep about 50 percent of excess weight loss after their surgery.

- Your hormones might adjust from a large weight loss, and this increases testosterone and improves metabolism.

- You could be able to get rid of your medicines used to treat high cholesterol or high blood pressure.

- You will eliminate or improve type 2 diabetes.

- You will absorb not as many calories from food. This is the result of bypassed intestines.

- You will give sick if you eat too many carbs or sugar. This is called dumping syndrome.

- You are not going to be able to eat huge meals. This is due to the restricted stomach size.

- You will lose weight. Within the first year and a half, you will lose approximately 70 percent of your body weight.
    - Research has shown up to a 77.5 percent of excess weight was lost 18 months after their procedure.

You will find exercise to be easier once you lose weight and you don't have to take as many medications as before. There is a possibility of losing more than average weight if you can learn to eat healthier and establish a regular exercise routine.

After your procedure, you will feel better, have more energy, and gain confidence. Studies have shown about 95 percent of all patients have reported a better quality of life for one year after surgery.

You have finally made it all the way to surgery. You have done your physician supervised diet, nutrition consults, psych evaluation, and lived through the liquid diet.

You will not be able to eat the night before. You will need to relax. Relax in a hot bath. Concentrate on why you need to have this procedure done. It is normal to have second thoughts and feel scared.

Surgery Day

You can't drink or eat anything the day of your procedure. This includes coffee or water unless you get permission from your anesthesiologist or surgeon. Once at the hospital, you will have paperwork to fill out including consent forms and be admitted. You will meet with the pre-op staff, your circulation nurse, and the anesthesiologist. If you are worried or have questions, there is no reason to be afraid to ask.

You will put on a hospital gown. To prevent blood clots from happening you will be asked to wear special socks. Many facilities will give you some medicine for anxiety. They will insert an IV into you, normally in the arm so intravenous fluids, antibiotics, and medicines can be given. This gives them a direct path straight into the bloodstream. The IV stays until you get discharged.

The operating room staff will put pads on your chest so they can keep track of your heart rate once you get into the operating room. They will administer anesthesia through your IV, and you will have a mask of oxygen placed over your face. They will ask you to count backward from ten. When you wake up, you will be in recovery.

After Surgery

It's done! The worst is done. The hard part begins.

The type of incision will determine how long it will take you to recover. If your procedure was done laparoscopically, you will probably stay in the hospital anywhere from two to three days. If the procedure was an open one your hospital stay and recovery might be longer.

The incision area will be sore after surgery. Pain is managed easily with medicine while you are in the hospital. You will stand and walk the day of your surgery. This helps to get rid of the gas that was used to inflate your abdomen in surgery. You will walk around at the minimum of three times each day after your surgery.

Most hospitals will insert a pain pump in the patient that lets them control their pain medication. You just press a button that pushes the pain medicine into your IV. This way you don't have to call a nurse and wait.

After your surgery, your surgeon will come check on you. They will also come by before your release. You need to understand all of the discharge instructions and any medicines or prescriptions that you will need at home.

Returning Home

Being home will be good. It can also be scary. You will be yourself.

When you begin to feel pain, take your medicine. There will be soreness. It may hurt more before it begins to feel better. Your doctor will prescribe medicine for your pain. Don't wait until you are home to get it. Ask a friend to pick it up for you. Take the medicine the way the doctor prescribed it. You might experience some constipation from the pain medicine. The instructions you received when you were discharged should tell you what to do to relieve your constipation.

You are going to need to walk when you can just don't do too much. You will feel extremely tired. You have just survived surgery and haven't had any solid food for several weeks. Take it easy for a couple of weeks. Walk around when you can.

Consume lots of water. Dehydration is bad after surgery. We get most of our water from the food we eat. Since you can't eat food, you are going to have to watch your intake of water to keep from getting dehydrated. Fill a bottle with how much water you are going to consume in a day's time and begin taking tiny sips. You absolutely CANNOT use straws when you consume water. You might consume too large of an amount and too fast. You could also swallow air which will put your stomach under pressure. Take tiny baby sips. NO STRAWS.

You might think you are going to start exercising immediately, helping around the house, organizing things, and cleaning the house. You must get your sleep. You are going to be tired. You have an eternity to get your house cleaned and organized. For the first few weeks, just plan on getting rest.

Sleeping in a recliner might be easier on you. A little bit of an incline might help with your stomach pain. It might also lessen the chance of getting heartburn. Use more pillows to prop yourself up with if you can't use a recliner.

You need to cough to expand your lungs and expel any fluids that might still be in your lungs after surgery. You have had surgery and coughing will hurt. Most doctors will suggest that you use a cough pillow. When you need to cough, just hold the pillow against your stomach. This will prevent any large movements of the stomach and reduces pain.

Follow the instructions you received at discharge. You shouldn't lift anything that weighs over 15 pounds for a minimum of six to seven weeks. Remember to walk. Increase the amount as your body will allow it. Try going up stairs when you think you will be able to do it, just take it easy. If something causes pain or is too hard, just stop.

You cannot get in a bathtub to soak. You will have to wait until after your follow-up appointment before you can shower. You need to make sure your incisions stay clean and have the time to heal. Redness around the incision is normal. Foul odors, pus, and drainage need to reported to your surgeon as soon as possible.

Your next appointment will be a week following the procedure. Your staples will get removed at this appointment. You will have another appointment a month later. The third a month after that. Many doctors will want to see you again in four months. The next will be six months after that. This will be a year after surgery was done. These times are just approximate. Each doctor will have their own schedules, or you might just need more visits.

Go to all of your appointments. Ask questions, talk about any problems you might be having. Your surgeon can't help if you can't be honest with them.

Once your annual checkup is done, your doctor is going to follow up with you at least one time a year. There will be blood work done and prescription refills during these appointments. The blood tests will let the doctors know if you are nutrient deficient.

Stretching Your Stomach

Absolutely. The stomach is comprised of tissues that constantly move to make room for what we consume. This stretching could be responsible for the full feeling we get after meals.

When you eat a lot, your stomach is going to stretch out and it will contract at a later time. Constantly eat large meals will cause you to think that you need a big meal to feel full. You could get into a cycle of eating until you are full and not letting your stomach contact before you eat again. You will begin to feel as if you have to consume even more to be full.

Here are some ways to keep you from stretching your stomach after surgery:

- Chew well and eat slowly.
- Don't drink while you eat. Both food and liquid will go to your stomach. Separate food and liquids by 30 minutes.
    - o Do not drink beverages that are carbonated. Bubbles will put pressure on your stomach.
- Learn to just eat a meal that has been predetermined and is appropriate for the time you have been out of surgery.
    - o You are consuming way too much food if what is on your plate is bigger than your fist.

Weight Loss to Expect

After gastric bypass surgery, you might lose between 60 and 80 percent of your extra weight. This will occur in the first 18 months. You are at risk to regain weight after your surgery. When compared to other treatment for the morbidly obese, gastric bypass has the best success.

Gastric bypass can help you get your weight to a healthy level. Once you get it where you want it, it is on you to keep it off. Here are some habits to help you after surgery:

- Get family members to start eating healthier.
- Join forums, make friends.
- Go to support groups.
- See your surgeon as recommended. It is amazing how many don't go back to their doctors after six months.
- Keep a journal on what you eat.
- Exercise three to five times each week.
- Eat three small healthy meals each day.

Lap Band patients have a weight loss of about 50 percent of the extra weight. People who have the gastric sleeve procedure can lose around 60 percent of their extra weight. Some might get lucky and lose 70 percent.

Saggy Skin

Losing a significant amount of weight fast can cause loose or sagging skin. It doesn't matter what caused the person to lose the weight. Anyone can get sagging skin if they lose weight too fast when they are morbidly obese. This will happen. You can have the skin removed if you need to.

Insurance will sometimes cover these.

As you grew, your skin stretched. Skin is full of elasticity but it won't completely shrink to fit over your new smaller body.

How old you are can factor in on how saggy the skin will get. Younger patient's skin has a lot more elasticity. The skin will lose elasticity as we get older. Younger patients haven't been overweight for as long. Their skin can bounce back faster.

The amount of weight that is lost will play a role. You are going to have saggy skin if you lose two to three hundred pounds. If the weight loss is around 50 to 100 pounds, you won't have as much saggy skin. If you are young, you might not have much loose skin at all.

This all seems fairly obvious, but this is very important. Setting the right expectations will help your happiness and satisfaction after your surgery. This procedure can improve health problems that go along with being obese. This is not cosmetic surgery.

These things can help to reduce but it will not get rid of all the saggy skin:

- Use sunscreen every time you go outside. Sun damages the skin and reduces elasticity.
- Eat vegetables and fruits.
- Stretch. Calisthenics and yoga will help build lean muscles and can make you look more toned.
- Use weights to exercise.
- Moisturize.
- Stay hydrated. Drink water to keep your skin healthy.

If you tried all of these and still have sagging skin that you don't like, it might require cosmetic surgery to fix. If it can't be determined to be medically necessary, your insurance will not cover it. If you have enough skin to cause skin rashes or infections, then you have a good chance of getting this problem taken care of. In 2013, surgeons performed close to 42,000 operations to correct body contours like reshaping of stomachs, thighs, arms, and breasts for patients that lost large amounts of weight. These types of operations can cost the very least $4,000 and go up from there.

Emotional Changes

After gastric bypass surgery, there will be some emotional changes. Depression can be caused by imbalances in testosterone, progesterone, and estrogen. Rapid weight loss can change the balance of thyroid production, estrogen, and testosterone.

This could be a good change since the increase in thyroid hormone could give the patient with hypothyroidism more energy. Losing weight quickly after surgery might change the estrogen and testosterone levels. These changes in hormones can create many difficult emotions. Regret, feeling hopeless, anger, and depression are common within the first year.

Getting yourself prepared for these changes can reduce the problems they cause. Having friends and family prepared and find a group to join can help lessen these problems. With time, your emotions and hormones will stabilize.

Some people have this surgery and don't experience any emotional problems.

Risks

The risks involved with surgery need to be weighed carefully but the benefits of gastric bypass are wonderful. Vomiting and nausea are not true complications but are common after surgery. They will typically resolve over time and with eating right. If you follow the supplement and vitamin regimen, then the chances of getting nutritional deficiencies are rare.

Death can result if major complications arise. Death after surgery extremely rare. The death rate is the same as having gallbladder surgery.

Pulmonary Embolism

When a blood clot forms after surgery and travels to your lungs, is called pulmonary embolism. It stops the right gas/blood exchange. You could have symptoms that include rapid heart rate, fainting, shock, shortness of breath, chest pain, and death. These instances are battled with blood thinners. You might need to have surgery or thrombolytics if the condition becomes life threatening. Thrombolytics are medicines that help break up bigger clots.

Staple Line Leaks

If the tissue that holds the staples breaks apart or if the staples were to fall out, it can cause leaks. This means that what is in your stomach or bowels can leak into your abdomen. If the leaks are found early, they can be repaired. You might have symptoms like fever, faster heart rate, and severe pain.

Surgeons can check for leaks two different ways. One test uses air and the doctor looks for bubbles. Another uses dye and looks for dye in the abdomen. If the leak is minor, it can be treated by resting the stomach and being fed through an IV. Surgery might be needed if the leak is severe.

Obstruction in the Bowel

An obstruction in the small bowel might happen after surgery. It could happen years later. You could have symptoms that include vomiting, swelling, and pain in the abdomen. A diagnosis could be made by either surgery or having a CAT scan. Treatment could require surgery.

Other Risks

Pregnancy

Women who are still able to get pregnant, need to wait a year and a half after they have surgery before they even think about getting pregnant.

Nausea

People who have this type of surgery usually have some nausea. You have a 70 percent chance of experiencing this. If you don't stick to your diet the doctor gives you, can cause nausea. Chewing your food thoroughly, not drinking while eating, eating the right things will reduce the chances of nausea.

Dehydration

When fluids are depleted, dehydration can occur. Sipping liquids throughout the day is the easiest way to prevent dehydration. The first week, when all you can do is drink water, is the most important time. Fill a 64-ounce bottle with water and sip slowly.

Indigestion

If you have pain in the upper part of your stomach, then you have a case of indigestion. Staying away from greasy foods and drinking lots of water is the best way to treat it. Antacids can be taken if changing your diet doesn't help your condition. Before you self-medicate, talk with your surgeon.

Infections at the Wound Site

Infections at the incision site can range from one and a half percent to 20 percent. It could be due to the technique that was used during surgery. If it gets treated early, antibiotics can help cure the infection. Open procedures have a higher risk.

Ulcers

There is a risk of developing ulcers after gastric bypass surgery. People who take certain medicines and smokers are at a higher risk of getting ulcers. At your discharge, you should have gotten a list that included medications to stay away from. DON'T SMOKE. Smoking increases the risk of ulcers. Here is are some medications that you will not be able to take. This is not a comprehensive list:

- Pepto-Bismol

- Motrin

- Excedrin

- Ibuprofen

- Alka-Seltzer

Other Possible Complications

Range in severity and could include gastric reflux, internal hernias, tissue ischemia, strictures, and many more.

What Does This Mean

This type of surgery is safe. The first thirty days after surgery the complication rate is around 5.9 percent. The risk of death is just like having any other surgical procedure like having your gallbladder removed.

Gastric bypass surgery has been well studied and is a great way to treat morbid obesity. Newer procedures to help the morbidly obese are out there. They don't have enough data, safety profile, and their results don't compare to gastric bypass. Gastric bypass is still the best procedure for losing weight and all candidates for bariatric surgery need to think about it.

Decide if Gastric Bypass is for you

Gastric bypass might be for you if:

- You want to make a lifestyle change to keep the weight off.
- You are ready to change how you eat.
- You know the benefits and risks
- You are an adult who is obese with a BMI of 40 or more, and you have a condition like a type 2 diabetes

Serious health problems related to obesity include:

- Sleep apnea
- Type 2 diabetes
- High cholesterol
- High blood pressure

Teens aren't a candidate for a gastric bypass unless they are morbidly obese, have a condition that is related to their weight, and have a body mass index of over 35.

If you don't meet any of these requirements, you could still qualify for a different procedure called Gastric Balloon.

Types of Surgery

When you undergo weight loss surgery, the surgeon will make changes to you small intestine or stomach or possibly both. Here are the methods they use:

Duodenal Switch: This surgery is complicated. It will remove a lot of the stomach and uses a sleeve to bypass the majority of the small intestines. This limits how much food you are able to consume. This means that your body won't be able to absorb the nutrients you need from the food you eat. This means that you won't be getting the right amounts of minerals and vitamins that you need.

Gastric Sleeve: This surgery will remove the majority of the stomach and will leave just a narrow section of the upper portion of the stomach referred to as a gastric sleeve. The surgery might curb the hunger hormone ghrelin to help you eat less.

Adjustable Gastric Band: With this surgery, the surgeon will put a small band around the upper part of the stomach. This band has a little balloon inside of it that can control how loose or tight the band is. This will limit how much food can move into the stomach. This is a laparoscopic surgery.

Gastric Bypass: Some doctors refer to this as Roux-en-Y gastric bypass or RYGB. The surgeon will leave a tiny part of the stomach, referred to as the pouch. This pouch doesn't hold much food. This makes you eat less. The food you consume bypasses most of the stomach and goes straight to the small intestines. This surgery is done by making several small incisions and using a camera to see inside. They can also do a mini-bypass. This procedure is similar and also done laparoscopically.

Electric Implant: This system works similarly to a pacemaker. It delivers electrical pulses to the vagus nerve that travels between the stomach and brain. This nerve will tell the brain that the stomach is full. The Maestro Rechargeable System is implanted into the abdomen. There is a remote control that adjusts it from outside the body. It isn't widely available yet, and the weight loss results aren't as impressive as gastric bypass surgery. It might not replace the need for gastric bypass. It might be an option for severely overweight people who need help losing weight down to a point where it will be safe for them to have gastric bypass. It can also be used for people who need help keeping their post-op weight under control. It would be worth talking about with your doctor.

With any weight loss surgery, you must focus on eating healthy and becoming active.

Benefits

After surgery, many people will lose weight for anywhere from 18 to 24 months. After this, many will begin to regain some weight, but never all of it.

Any medical conditions that are related to obesity that you might have will usually improve after surgery. Conditions like diabetes could improve very quickly. High blood pressure might take longer.

It can also help with:

- Sleep apnea
- Cholesterol problems
- High cholesterol
- Cardiovascular disease
- Venous stasis disease
- Bone and joint disease like osteoarthropathy
- Depression
- Migraines
- Pseudotumor cerebri
- Gastroesophageal reflux disease
- Non-alcoholic fatty liver disease
- Asthma

- Obstructive sleep apnea
- Stress urinary incontinence
- Polycystic ovarian syndrome
- Pregnancy
- Type 2 diabetes
- Mortality reduction
- Improves quality of life
- Metabolic syndrome

Side Effects and Risks

The side effects that are most common are dizziness, increased gas, excessive sweating, diarrhea, bloating, vomiting, and nausea.

Serious side effects might include blood clots in the legs that might move to the lungs or heart, leaks from your stitches, infections, and bleeding. Most patients won't get these.

Problems lasting for a long time will depend on what type of surgery you have. The most common issue with gastric bypass is dumping syndrome. This is where food moves extremely quickly through the small intestines. You might have symptoms of diarrhea, faintness, sweating, weakness, and nausea after you eat. You won't be able to eat sweets without feeling weak. This could happen in about 50 percent of the people who had gastric bypass surgery. If you can avoid foods that are high in sugar and replace them with fiber rich foods, it might help to prevent this problem.

Gallstones might form when you lose weight very quickly. You doctor might recommend taking supplemental bile salts for about six months after your surgery to help prevent this.

If the surgery made it harder on your body to get nutrients from food, you will need to be sure you are getting plenty of nutrients.

Nutritional deficiencies and rapid weight loss can hurt a fetus. Women of childbearing years are typically told to wait until their weight has stabilized before trying to get pregnant.

Things Your Doctor Might Not Tell You

If you have been thinking about it, you are probably getting a lot of post- and pre-op guidance from people you trust. For many who undergo this procedure, life after surgery is full of surprises. The surprises are almost like an old western: the good, the bad, and the embarrassing. If you are serious about bariatric surgery, here are some thing you need to know that your doctor might forget.

Depression and obesity are linked. Most patients do feel an improvement in well-being after the surgery. The feelings of depression can get worse for others. Researchers from Yale did a study where 13 percent of the patients that were studied had an increase in Beck Depression Inventory for six to 12 months following the surgery. This is a rating that measures social functioning, self-esteem, and eating disorder behaviors. This time frame is the most important time to check for depression and other symptoms.

You will poop a lot more. Most patients who have gastric bypass surgery will have times of extreme diarrhea called dumping syndrome sometime after the surgery. This happens due to eating the wrong foods like dairy, fats, fried foods, and refined sugars. You could have symptoms that include active audible bowel sounds, cramping, nausea, wanting to lie down, lightheadedness, flushing, and sweating. Sound horrible? Well, that isn't all: embarrassing gas, constipation, and loose stools are the other bowel-related problems post-surgery.

It can raise the risk of alcohol abuse. One study checked patients of gastric bypass surgery at one, three, six, and 24-month intervals after their surgery and saw that the risk for alcohol abuse was higher. This might be due to patients having higher peak levels. They reach these levels quicker after surgery.

You need a gym membership. Most doctors talk to their patients about the right post-surgery diet to help with weight-loss. That is the most important lifestyle change that patients have to do. When a patient gets cleared by their doctor to introduce exercise into their daily routine. Start slow and gradually work up to an hour of exercise six days each week. This is best for helping with weight loss success. So, don't think that you are going to get off easy. Surgery is not a quick fix.

Say goodbye to soda. Carbonated beverages are forbidden since the introduce air into the belly. It creates gas that puts undue pressure on the stomach and will make it expand unnecessarily. It essentially undoes what the surgery does. Drink water since dehydration is the main reason that patients get readmitted to the hospital.

It can cause a strain on a marriage. Massive physical transformations could lead to many emotional changes that can affect both you and your relationship. One study showed an increase in divorce rates among couples who had one member undergo gastric bypass surgery. If this is going to happen, it will happen in the first year after the surgery. You might need to think about looking for emotional guidance for you and your spouse in addition to your medical care. You can seek counseling by joining a support group or finding a therapist. This can help with the negative effects on the relationship.

The risks are low when you compare them with doing nothing. Weight loss surgery has a bad reputation for being risky. Procedures have improved and are much safer now. The chances of having any major complications are about 4.3 percent. The risks of staying obese are stroke, diabetes, heart disease, and possibly death. These are incredibly more dangerous.

Many patients say they would have it done again. Success is a long-term project for people who have this procedure done. Many people say if they went back in time, they would have the surgery done all over again. Many people said that after their surgery and weight loss they felt a lot better. They are also more active and don't have as many medicines to take to help with their complications from being overweight. These can all improve anyone's quality of life.

Out of Pocket Costs

The following will look at what you might have to spend if you have insurance that doesn't or won't pay for this type of surgery.

Let's first compare what the costs are depending on what country you live in:

- Australia - $17,000
- Canada - $20,000
- Costa Rica - $12,500
- India - $10,400
- Mexico - $7, 400
- Thailand - $10,500
- United States - $24,000 ranges from $15,000 in Arkansas to $57,000 in Alaska

The out-of-pocket cost will depend on different factors that include:

- If your procedure is laparoscopic or open – open will cost about $2,500 more than laparoscopic.

- What hospital you choose to have your surgery in.

- If you have insurance or not. If the hospital and surgeon are covered by insurance, a discount has been agreed upon that allow the hospital and surgeon to participate with your company's network.

- If you can get some financing for some of the costs.

- Certain fees your surgeon and other hospital staff charge for various services.

The averages about include total cost that incurs during the surgery. Some surgeons will include pre-op costs in their quotes.

The above prices don't include post-op costs that are based on your specific conditions.

Surgery costs might be further complicated by:

- Different hospitals, same surgeon: Some surgeons have what they call operating privileges at more than one hospital. Since costs at hospitals can vary widely – even in the same city and it doesn't matter about quality – ask your surgeon if you can choose a certain hospital.

- Other discounts: More discounts could be offered for paying your bill upfront. Ask your doctor is they give discounts that you can take advantage of.

- Self-Pay discounts: Many weight loss surgery clinics offer some sort of self-pay discount or a payment plan in case you don't have insurance, or if your insurance doesn't cover the procedure. You just need to ask them.

Recovery

Recovery time from having gastric bypass surgery will include:

- Timeline: Between four and six weeks for full recovery
    - o Hospital stay will be between one and three days
    - o Time from work will be one to three weeks
- Pain: Just like any other laparoscopic surgery, it is managed with medication
- Diet: Will be a slow transition from clear liquids to solid foods
- Activity: Will be a slow transition to get back to regular exercise and activities
- Challenges: You will face some challenges like sagging skin, short-term hair loss, kidney stones, gallstones, possible dental issues, weight gain if you cheat on the diet, digestive issues, dumping syndrome.

Preparing for Your Surgery

Being prepared for your weight loss surgery will help you:

- Help you keep the weight off forever
- Increase how much weight you will lose
- Lessen having complications
- Save money
- Reduce stress

Here are some reasons why you should lose weight while getting ready for your surgery:

1. Less likely to have complication during surgery.
2. Lose more weight after surgery.

For every one percent of weight loss before surgery, you can lose about 1.8 percent more weight in one year.

Patients that had lost weight in excess of five percent had shorter operating times. Basically, lower weight will make it easier for the surgeons to do the procedure. Spending less time in the operating room lowers your risk of complications.

Other studies found a direct link between weight loss before surgery and the number of complications. The more weight a patient can lose before surgery, the less likely they are the have complications.

Another reason for preparing for surgery early is getting rid of bad habits. It takes time to break habits. Weight loss surgery won't work if you can't change your habits.

If you begin to eat after surgery, the way you ate before, you will gain all the weight back, and you will have a relapse in your health problems associated with obesity.

A runner would never try to do a marathon without getting in shape for months before; a bypass surgery patient should never go into surgery without being prepared.

The sooner you begin to prepare for surgery; you will be able to establish good habits that are needed to achieve your health improvement and weight loss goals that you have already set.

Logistics, Payment, and Medical Care Checklist:

- Begin to work with your surgical team: From financing to insurance considerations that are required like pre-op tests and pre-op instructions that are specific to you. There are different issues that your surgeon will be able to address while you are preparing for your surgery. Learn about options or go to a seminar, to get a better handle and what you need to expect and learn how to work with the team.

- Understand the payment and savings opportunities and options
    o If you have insurance, confirm the benefits and figure out what they require.
    o If you don't have insurance and aren't able to pay in full up front, you will need to arrange financing.
- Schedule pre-op testing, physicals, and consultations to make sure you are a candidate for surgery.

- Start and plan your diet plan that will be supervised by your surgeon. Figure out what medical history and paperwork you are going to need to be able to move forward. For example, psychological evaluation, medical records, letter of medical clearance, and letter of medical necessity.

- After all the tests have been done, and you have completed all paperwork and meet all requirements, the surgeon's office will make sure that you are able to proceed with the surgery and will get the pre-authorization from the insurance company if needed.

- Your surgeon might make you do other steps or attend other meetings. They will guide you after a pre-approval.

Lifestyle Changes Checklist

To achieve your goals of improving your health and weight loss after surgery, you have to begin living like you had already had the surgery three months ago.

- Start eating for your health and not for pleasure and flavor – Your stomach will be smaller after surgery, and this will prevent the body from processing the amount of food you are used to eating. This is wonderful for weight loss but horrible for getting the nutrition that your body needs to work right. If you just eat junk food, you won't get the nutrients that are needed after surgery. You will suffer a horrible side effect of malnutrition and possibly dumping syndrome.

  o Begin thinking about food as fuel for the body. When you eat, see how your body reacts to the food. Begin watching for cues for when you feel hungry and full. Eat mindfully. Don't eat while watching TV or at your desk. Work on eliminating reactive energy. Don't eat when you feel stressed, tired, or bored. Don't use food to cope with emotional problems. This is going to be hard to do while preparing for your surgery but should get a bit easier after surgery. You will be able to eat all sorts of things after you retrain your taste buds. Your taste buds will change after surgery. The things you enjoyed eating won't appeal to you anymore.

- Eat a lot of protein. Protein is necessary for weight loss because it helps you feel fuller quicker and for longer. It also helps you keep muscles during the rapid weight loss after surgery.

- Watch portion sized, chew each bite thoroughly, and eat slowly. Feeling full will take about 20 to 30 minutes to get to your brain. Chewing thoroughly and eating slowly will help you stay in touch with your body so that you won't overeat and stretch your smaller stomach. By practicing eating this way before surgery will help you lose the weight.

- Begin taking multi vitamins. Since gastric bypass surgery, patients can't absorb nutrients because of the changes to the digestive system and from not eating as much. You will need to take supplements. Begin implementing this into your routine before surgery. Talk with your doctor about what multivitamins they want you to take.

- Don't drink while you eat. After surgery, you must wait 30 minutes before drinking anything. Liquids can flush the food straight through your smaller stomach and cause you to feel hungry faster and cause you to gain your weight back.

  o After surgery, you won't have much space in your stomach for fluids and food. You might get dehydrated or malnourished if you don't drink and eat separately. This is a very important step especially when you are still healing.

- Get rid of the sugary drinks and consume more water. If you don't have fluid restrictions, begin to drink 64 ounces of water each day. Drinking water during the months you are preparing for weight loss surgery will help patients by feeling full, keeping yourself hydrated and keeping your kidneys flushed out, so you don't develop kidney stones.

- Be careful drinking coffee. Small amounts of coffee are fine by staying away from the calories from cream and sugar. To help ease the transition, high-caffeine tea with honey is a good alternative.

- Stop consuming alcohol. Because of changes to your digestive system, alcohol will have a different effect on the body. It is going to be easier to get drunk. This means that you will possibly give into good cravings. Consuming alcohol after surgery can cause your blood sugar to go crazy and result in weight gain.

- Exercise more. Begin slow, do what you enjoy, begin moving. You should be able to move for 20 to 30 minutes every day. This reduces the risk of complications developing during surgery. It will help with weight loss before surgery, and it gets you into the habit that leads to weight loss in the long run.

- Stop smoking. Smoking will increase the risk of getting blood clots during surgery. These risks can stay with you for about six weeks after you last inhale smoke.

- Begin going to support groups. It is important to hear other's experiences. Other patients can give you insights that your surgical team can't provide. This also lets you build relationships that will help you succeed after surgery. Ask your surgeon for names and locations of support groups.

These changes are not going to be easy; this is why you need to start early. Be patient. Practice forgiveness and self-management. When you begin to change your routine in the weeks and months, you are preparing for weight loss surgery. The adjustment will get easier and easier.

Two Weeks Out Checklist

Two weeks before your surgery, you have completed all your pre-op tests, physical, and anything else your insurance company or surgeon has asked you to do. You should have gotten your authorization from the insurance for the payment to the hospital and surgeon.

You are drinking and eating just like you have already had the surgery.

You are exercising or walking for 20 minutes each day.

Your surgery time and date are set, and you know when to arrive at the hospital.

In the couple of weeks that lead up to your surgery, you will be seeing the pre-surgery department at the hospital for EKGs, blood work, and any other tests or instructions. You will see the surgeon for a pre-op physical, consents, and any last-minute details.

The night before you won't be able to drink or eat anything after midnight.

Here is a checklist of things you need to have before the surgery:

- Take time off from work. You are going to need time to figure out what your body will be able to tolerate, adjust to your stomach, and time to recover, so about four to six week is normal.

- Talk to your doctor about getting your post-op prescriptions before your surgery. By doing this, you won't need to worry about getting any prescriptions filled during your recovery.

- Have child care figured out?

- Someone will need to take you to the hospital and bring you home.

- You are going to need someone with you for the first week after your surgery. This person needs to be with you 24/7. Be sure they have asked for time off from their jobs as well.

- Begin preparing the vitamins and food that you are going to eat after surgery. You could make a shopping list for someone else to get these items for you, so they will be at home waiting on you.

- Make sure you have comfortable sleeping arrangements because you are going to be sore after your surgery.

- Comfortable items to think about for the hospital stay and your ride home:

  o Hygiene items, shampoo, comb, toothbrush, toothpaste, soap, other.

  o Clothes

  o Entertainment

  o CPAP machine

  o Sleep aids

  o Other

You might need to tackle some issues to get yourself mentally prepared for surgery. Here are some tips that will help get you emotionally ready for your surgery:

1. Begin with expectations that are realistic

You will not wake up thin after your surgery. You might leave the hospital weighing more due to fluid build-up. Remember that surgery isn't the immediate answer to weight loss; instead, it is a tool that will help you with your weight loss. This tool is your smaller stomach.

You should use it to take about six months to lose about half of your weight. Then you might hit a plateau. It might take another year to actually get to your weight loss goal.

Your weight loss is a journey that takes effort and time. Knowing the process will help you not to give up and stay on track.

2. Don't try this alone

You need a good support system if you are seriously thinking about surgery.

Talk to your primary care provider and other family member or friends to help you with your long-term goals. Get someone to keep track of your weight-loss milestones and keep you motivated.

The thought of bariatric surgery is scary for most people. It might help if you take baby steps. Instead of trying to do everything at one time, check out your options and pick just a couple of resources. Here are some first steps you can look at:

- Talk with your doctor about starting a weight-loss program
- Consider and investigate joining a support group
- Watch online seminars about it
3. Confront and recognize food addictions

If you are addicted to food, this will need to be addressed before you have surgery. Getting a smaller stomach with bariatric surgery isn't going to fill your emotional needs that eating does.

Most people use food to deal with stress. This is short-term to manage problems. It also creates more issues. Broadening your perspectives can help you to see how valuable making healthier food choices and limiting how much you eat.

You must be at a point where you want to feel better, want to change and do other activities instead of eating all the time. For some, they must want to focus on the long-term goals for their lives instead of the food they will be eating for their next meal. Others get motivated by the daily illness and pain that comes with excess weight.

Learning to manage your food is crucial after surgery to keep your weight loss because:

- A healthy diet is crucial. You can't graze on junk food. This will sabotage your ability to lose weight.

- You must eat slowly. A small meal should take you 20 minutes to eat.

- Your food intake is going to be restricted drastically, especially in the first few months.

4. Depression might become an issue

Gastric bypass surgery is around 80 percent effective. It will take focus and time to keep the weight off. Your emotional energy needs to be working to help your efforts.

After the surgery, your body will be recovering, and eating is physically restricted. If you have depression, it will be harder to keep on track, especially if you have a food addiction.

Work with counselors and doctors to maintain and develop a positive attitude.

5. Know the risks about other addictions

Tobacco and alcohol addictions can hinder your efforts to lose weight without or with surgery.

Alcohol is very high in calories and will reduce your inhibitions. This will make you more susceptible to eating more than you should. You will also feel its intoxicating effects quicker after you have surgery. Consuming just one alcoholic beverage could put you over the legal blood alcohol limit.

Tobacco use will increase the risk of ulcers, respiratory problems, and surgical complications. Patients who start smoking again after surgery could develop post- surgical stomach irritations or ulcers.

Life Changing

Gastric bypass surgery could change your life. You can use this tool to provide you with sustained relief if you are overweight.

The benefits of weight loss through gastric bypass surgery might include:

- Alleviation of other medical problems like gallbladder disease, pregnancy complications, metabolic syndrome, and more.
- Improved fertility
- Relief from pain in the joints
- Elimination of sleep apnea
- Depression relief
- Cardiovascular health will improve
- Type 2 diabetes can go into long-term remission

Focus on what contributed to your weight gain. What has caused you to not be able to make changes? Focus on how ready you are for change in your life now. Begin keeping a journal of all the motivational and healthy changes you are making. Create a network of caring, positive people. Find different ways to cope with emotional eating. Surgery is just the beginning of your weight-loss journey. You have a lot of work ahead of you. Making lifestyle changes is going to take time. Take small steps. Make realistic goal. Above all stay positive.

Eating after the Surgery

Gastric bypass surgery can save your life. You are going to lose weight. You will look and feel better. You need to change your diet to be successful.

It might sound simple, but it really isn't. Get ready to struggle. You have spent most of your life reinforcing and building bad habits. Those must change.

Getting into the habit of eating right before you have surgery and sticking with it is important. Here's why:

- The higher your BMI is before surgery, the higher risk of developing complications. Getting on track with your diet before surgery will reduce your risks and bring down your BMI.

- It gives you the nutrients and energy it will need to heal correctly from surgery. It will help your body function properly during your extreme weight loss.

- It will help avoid surgery complications in the long run while boosting weight loss and keeping it off.

Knowing what you can't and can eat is the beginning of a healthy diet. What you eat for the first five weeks after surgery is very important. Here are two reasons why:

1. Safety. Eating the wrong foods will put pressure on your stomach while it is trying to heal.

2. Replacing your bad eating with new healthier habits.

The convention might tell you to live it up since you are having surgery. In reality, you need to have the opposite mentality.

From the moment you seriously began to consider weight loss surgery, you diet habits must change forever. Look at the months that are leading up to surgery as a test. You are in training to discipline and learn the motivation it is going to take to get to your goals.

The right surgeon will help you. Finding a good doctor and learning about the nutritionist or dietitian that they have on staff is part of the process. The dietitian will do a consult about your diet history and help you understand the kind of eater you are.

They will point you to the bariatric treatment that will help your habits. They will get you on the appropriate diet.

Before most bariatric insurance providers will approve your surgery, they make you go through a medically-supervised program.

A low carb/high protein diet is needed for three reasons:

1. Shrinks your liver

2. Promotes healing

3. Reduces bleeding

To make sure you are ready for surgery. DO NOT go out and have one last huge unhealthy meal. Don't sit around and binge on your favorite foods because you know you can't have these foods anymore.

Pre-op Diet

To reduce how much fat is in the spleen and liver, a preoperative liquid diet must be down seven to 14 days before your surgery. If you do not follow this diet, the surgery will have to be put off or canceled during the procedure.

It is so important it can't be stressed enough. You have already waited about six months or a year to get all the approvals. Don't let a diet stop you now.

If your liver is too large, the surgeon won't be able to see certain parts of your internal anatomy during the surgery. It will become unsafe to do the surgery. Surgery might be canceled or rescheduled for later.

Your dietitian or surgeon will put you on a pre-op diet a couple of weeks before your surgery. This diet will involve:

- Five to seven shakes each day as meal replacements. Low carb, high protein shakes are the best.

- Sugar-free beverages are okay.

- No carbonated or caffeinated drinks.

- Vegetable and V8 juices are fine.

- Broth or soup that doesn't have any food pieces in it can be eaten.

- Very thin cream of rice and cream of wheat can be eaten.

- Drink 64 to 96-ounces water each day.

- Some surgeons might allow a very small amount of vegetables a day.

- A couple servings of lean meat may be okay, but they must be approved by the dietician or surgeon.

All liquids and beverages need to be sipped extremely slowly. Beverages can't be drunk with meals. You must wait 30 minutes after you eat before you can drink anything.

Separating solids and liquids applies to after surgery, but it would be a good idea to start before your surgery.

During this phase, your body will hit ketosis. This will allow your body to use the fat it has stored for energy. This results in the fat in your liver will shrink a lot in a very short amount of time. Your diet is going to be low in carbs and high in protein. Here are some suggestions for meal replacement shakes:

- GNC Total Lean Shake 25
- Chike
- Unjury
- Isopure
- EAS Myoplex Light/Carb Control
- Bariatric Advantage

Consult your doctor about stopping some medicines before your surgery. The following medicines are usually stopped about a week before your surgery, and you might need to taper down the dose instead of just stopping them totally:

- Birth Control
- Replacement hormones
- Celebrex, Advil, Motrin, Aspirin, and other NSAIDs
- Anticoagulation medicines
- Steroids
- Coumadin

If you use a CPAP machine, you will need to bring it to the hospital. Purchase your supplements and vitamins in advance. Find good protein shakes.

You must stop smoking before your surgery. Smokers have more of a risk of complications and blood clots during and after surgery. Create a plan and implement it before the surgery.

- Do not drink or eat anything the day of your surgery.
- Resist doing a "Last Supper." A stomach that is empty is easier to work with.

Post-op Diet

When your surgery is done, a strict diet plan will need to be followed. You now have a smaller stomach. Your insides have been cut, re-routed, and moved around. You have staples in your stomach that need to heal completely. Some foods can disrupt this process, put stress on the staples, cause a leak. Large meals, carbonated beverages, fibrous foods can all lead to a staple leak. Don't risk having serious complications. Stick to your post-op diet.

There are four phases to this diet:

1. Clear liquids
2. Protein shakes and pureed foods
3. Soft foods
4. Solid foods

Week One/Phase One: Clear Liquids

After your surgery, you will be put on a diet plan. If you can follow their advice, it will help you heal and begin your permanent diet while keeping the side effects to a minimum. For the first week after surgery, you can only have clear liquids. You can consume an ounce or two every hour. Your dietician will figure out how long this will last and suggest some guidelines. Clear liquids will probably include the following:

- Sugar-free jello
- Fat-free broth
- Fat-free milk
- Water

You must stay well hydrated during this time. Some surgeons might want you to begin protein shakes within a few days after surgery. Stick to your surgeon's guidelines.

Weeks Two and Three/Phase Two: Protein Shakes and Pureed Foods

Your doctor will figure out when the second phase can begin. After drinking only clear liquids for a week, you will be allowed to begin consuming liquefied protein sources. This stage will usually last about a week.

Since your stomach is smaller, you should eat several small meals throughout the day. During this time, try to eat slowly. It should take you 30 minutes to eat every portion of food. Slowly eating your meals, and taking 30 minutes for each meal, needs to remain your goal through all these phases and after.

Your intake daily needs to be about 60 or 70 grams of protein from pureed fish or meat, egg whites, and protein shakes. You should drink 64 ounces of clear liquids. This isn't counting fluids from pureed foods.

Carbonated drinks, caffeine, sugar, and fat need to be avoided.

Here are some pureed protein sources that your doctor or dietitian might allow you to eat:

- Non-fat cottage cheese
- Non-fat soft cheese
- Egg whites
- Protein shakes

These food sources need to be pureed with fat-free broth, fat-free milk, or water. Water can't be consumed while eating the pureed foods. You shouldn't drink anything 30 minutes before and 60 minutes after.

Clear liquids need to be sipped slowly. Straws are forbidden as they can bring air to the stomach.

You will need to take some multivitamins that contain iron each day to prevent nutrient deficiencies. This needs to be in liquid or chewable form.

You will also need to a calcium citrate supplement. The amount that is recommended is usually two or three doses. Each dose will range between 400 and 600 milligrams. The calcium citrate supplements need to be separated from the multi vitamins by two hours. This is due to calcium and iron could interfere with each other's absorption.

Weeks Four and Five/Phase Three: Soft Foods

This stage allows you to very gradually reintroduce soft foods into the diet. This will last about one or two weeks.

If the food can be mashed with a spoon, knife, or fork, then it can be eaten. This phase of the diet will allow cooked vegetables and soft meats.

The nutrient goals are going to be the same. Consuming a half gallon of water and protein at around 70 grams. The serving sizes of protein need to be one to two ounces and eating three to six small meals.

This stage just like stage two will focus on lean protein sources.

Three servings of soft vegetable might be allowed. A tiny portion of fat might be permitted. This fat portion will be from a serving of avocado.

Recommended protein sources might include several of the following:

Eggs, Dairy, and Meat

- Tofu
- Non-fat cheese
- Non-fat cottage cheese
- Egg whites
- Fish
- Lean turkey
- Lean chicken

Vegetables

- Avocados
- Bananas
- Cucumbers
- Squash
- Tomatoes
- Green beans
- Carrots
- Potatoes

You are still going to need two multivitamins and two or three doses of calcium citrate. Remember to take these doses two hours apart.

Your dietitian might have you to take 1,000 IU of Vitamin D3 each day. This will probably be divided into two 500 IU doses. These can be taken with your calcium citrate. A dose of sublingual B12 might also be recommended. A weekly or monthly intranasal or injection is available for B12. Some dietitians might want you to take Vitamin B12 and D3 supplements in stage two.

Week Six/Phase Four: Solid Foods

Finally, solid food again. You have made it to this point, and you get to begin eating real food. This by no means allows you to eat whatever you want. This is the last phase. Go slow. Introducing foods too fast might cause dumping syndrome, heartburn, bloating, and painful gas. Wait a full day before you introduce any other new foods.

The goal needs to be reintroducing your body to healthy foods in little quantities. Continue to begin with soft food and wait until later for the more fibrous foods.

Your diet will consist of very little if any, refined sugars, limited amounts of grain, vegetables, and protein. You will eat this for the rest of your life.

Keep track of the amount of protein and make sure you are eating vegetables that are healthy as your carb source. Don't eat any junk carbs like chips, bread, rice, pasta, and refined sugar.

You can begin to lower the number of meals to three smaller meals each day. If you need to, you can drink protein shakes. Remember to take your supplements.

Your calorie intake is going to increase to between 1,000 and 1,500 each day. Don't force yourself. Eat what you can. There are some foods that the body just can't break down. These need to be added slowly and in little portions. Foods included are grapes, shellfish, pork, beef, beans, nuts, and corn.

Here are some tips to begin eating solid foods:

- Introduce one new food at a time. No more than one food each day until you can see how your body will react.

- Eat slow. Chew your food for 15 seconds for every bite.

- Separate food and water for 30 minutes.

- Remember to consume 64 ounces of water daily.

- Eat the protein first, vegetables next, and carbs last. These need to be fruits, or healthy grains and not any processed foods.

- Eat foods rich in nutrients. Don't consume processed and pre-packaged foods that have a lot of ingredients.

- Read the labels. Focus on foods that are low in carbs. The calorie to protein ration needs to be ten to one. When reading food labels, add a zero to the number of grams of protein. If that number is more than the total calories, then you might want to stay away from that food especially if you are trying to reach your protein goal.

Dumping Syndrome

The pylorus is a safety valve for your body. This doesn't let food go to the small intestines until gastric juices break it down. The surgery bypasses the pylorus. There may be times after your surgery that your stomach dumps its contents straight into the small intestines. We call this dumping syndrome. This occurs when fatty foods or sweets have been consumed too fast or too much of them. The stomach will dump the food into the small intestines before it gets broken down correctly. Dumping syndrome can cause increased heart rate, vomiting, dizziness, sweating, diarrhea, cramping, and nausea. These symptoms will wear off after a couple of hours. The experience of dumping is extremely unpleasant, and you will want to avoid it for the rest of your life.

Dumping syndrome will make you learn to eat right. You might just experience dumping syndrome if you don't eliminate or reduce carbs and refined sugars and eat small meals slowly. This will be the strongest motivator to keep away from unhealthy foods.

Early dumping is a form of dumping syndrome that will happen in about an hour and a half after you eat. The symptoms will include vomiting, bloating, dizziness, diarrhea, cramps, nausea, and sweating. Late dumping is another form that will occur more than an hour after you eat. This will have the same symptoms as early dumping. It might also include fainting and hunger.

The same guidelines that are in stage three are carried into this fourth and final stage. The protein intake, vitamin supplements, and liquids stay the same.

More vegetables and fruits, raw and cooked, can now be added to your diet. Small amounts of fat and incredibly small amounts of sugar can be added with caution. Caffeinated and carbonated beverages can be consumed in moderation.

Total calorie intake will be anywhere from 800 to 1,200. It can be raised up to 1,500 18 months after your surgery.

To help reduce dumping:

1. Stay away from refined sugars and carbs.
2. Eat slowly.
3. Chew each bite well.

Some foods are harder to digest and need to be eaten with caution:

- Beans
- Corn
- Whole grains
- Nuts
- Grapes
- Shellfish
- Pork
- Beef

You want to choose foods that are moderate to high in protein, moderate in good fats, and low in carbs.

Foods that have healthy fats:

- Coconut oil
- Nut butters
- Sardines
- Nuts
- Salmon
- Avocados

Some general guidelines to consider:

- Every meal should be the size of your fist.
- Introduce new foods slowly.
- Separate food and water by 30 minutes.
- Take vitamins and nutritional supplements.
- Eat out occasionally.
- Cut out fast food completely.
- Don't tempt yourself by filling your pantry with junk food.
- Eliminate or limit desserts.
- Shop for healthy foods.
- Involve the whole family in healthy eating decisions.
- Plan meals.
- Eat foods that are dense in nutrients.
- Stay away from whole milk
- Stay away from spicy and greasy foods
- Canned salmon and tuna.
- Choose lean meats.

Supplements and Vitamins

The size of your new stomach is going to restrict how much food you will be able to eat. Your bypassed intestines will reduce how many minerals and vitamins are absorbed from food. It will be necessary to take supplements and vitamins for your entire life after you have surgery.

Multivitamin

You will have to take a couple multivitamins during either the second or third phase of your diet plan. These will need to be taken with meals, and this will need to be continued for your entire life.

Calcium Citrate

This is another important supplement. It will need to be taken with meals but not when you take your multivitamin since the iron will keep the body from absorbing the calcium. Some dietitians and doctors might want you to begin this supplement in phase two others in the next phase.

Calcium carbonate doesn't absorb as good as calcium citrate.

Vitamin D3

You will begin taking Vitamin D3 either during phase two or three. They will tell you to take about 500 individual units two times a day. These can be taken at the same time as the calcium citrate.

Vitamin B12

Your digestive system can't process the right amounts of B12 after the surgery. It is recommended to take around 500 to 1,200 mcg of vitamin B12. Try to find the kind that you put under your tongue. By doing it this way, it gets absorbed into the bloodstream faster.

B12 can also be injected monthly. This can be done by your doctor at check-ups or you could do it yourself.

Iron

The duodenum absorbs iron. This part of the small intestine gets bypassed. Your body can't absorb the right amount of iron. The iron from multivitamins might not be enough. You might have to take an actual iron supplement. This holds true for females who are on their menstrual cycle.

Vitamin C helps your body absorb iron so it might be advisable to begin taking a supplement. Your doctor will determine the amount and type. Taking around 500 to 1,000 milligrams daily is what most patients get prescribed. The best bioavailable form of iron supplements are ferrous gluconate and ferrous fumarate.

Remember not to take iron when you take calcium as they will interfere with each other's absorption.

Exercise and Physical Activity

It is time to begin exercising. You really should have begun in stage two. Hiking, badminton, canoeing, aerobics, weight lifting, biking, running, walking, and dancing like a mad person can be added to your routine. Make sure you are exercising at least 30 minutes five to seven days a week. It doesn't matter how, just do it.

Do not lift anything heavier than ten pounds for about six weeks after your surgery. This can put pressure on your internal stitches and cause a hernia.

Tip for the Hard Times

Have you ever stopped to count how many times each week you eat away from home? If you are like the average American, you probably eat four or five commercially prepared meals each week from different places. This might sound like a lot but just think about it...How many times do you stop a Starbucks on your way to work? Do you grab lunch at the corner coffee shop? Order Italian or Chinese on nights you are too tired to cook? This isn't even counting special occasions or date nights.

When we eat food that isn't prepared in our kitchens, we are eating bigger portions and more calories. Studies have shown that we eat one to two hundred more calories per meal when we order food instead of cooking at home. Sometimes we find ourselves just too busy or don't have enough time to cook a meal at home. We have to find a balance by eating out less and making good choices when we do. People who are preparing for or have recovered from gastric bypass surgery, need to make smart choices to make sure they are getting the right amount of protein they need. Here are some tips to help pick the best and stay away from the worst selections on popular menus:

- Make sure you choose a balance of healthy fat, fiber, and protein that will fill you up and keep you from having blood sugar lows and highs.

- If you don't see anything on the menu, ask if you can create your own plate. Most restaurants will accommodate any dietary needs.

- Never drink your calories. Protein shakes or low-fat milk are exceptions to this rule. Beverages that are full of sugar like soda, specialty coffees, sports drinks, and juice need to be avoided.

- Order first at the table or office. We have a tendency to order like other we are with. Going first means that you will stick with your first healthy choice.

- The two main standards for weight loss and eating healthy are how much and what to eat. A couple high protein appetizers can make a satisfying meal. Some restaurants will allow postoperative adults to make choices from the children's menu or prepare half portions.

- Plan ahead. Check the menus online. If it is the day before or at breakfast, knowing what you are going to eat for dinner or lunch helps you plan your day.

Italian/Pizza

Having an occasional slice of pizza can be eaten in a healthy post-operative diet. The best pizza choice is a couple of slices of thin crust loaded with vegetables. Throw on some grilled chicken for protein, and you can indulge without completely derailing your efforts.

If you need to choose from a regular Italian menu, you might need to create your own entrée. Most restaurants will put their sauces or entrees over sautéed spinach or other vegetables instead of pasta. Stay away from cream sauces and anything that is fried. These will be too high in fat and calories. Look for entrees with broiled or grilled seafood, shrimp, or chicken. If you just absolutely can't stay away from the pasta, as for a small side order and eat it last. Better still, ask someone you are eating with for a couple bites of theirs.

Fast Food Restaurants

Depending on the chain, choices can vary. The best choices would be salads with grilled chicken and a half portion of low-fat dressing. Grilled fish or chicken sandwiches eaten without a bun. A cheeseburger or hamburger with onion, tomato, and lettuce without mayonnaise or sauces is always a good choice. Don't eat the bun and you will cut out 200 calories of empty carbs. It is best to stay away from anything fried or crispy, sauces like salad dressings, mayonnaise, honey mustard, and barbecue.

Southwest/Latin/Mexican

This cuisine can be challenging, but it can offer healthy options. The key is to stay away from the high-carb sides and choose vegetables and lean protein. Fajita platters without the tortillas and rice are filling and flavorful. Begin with any lean protein like flank steak, pork loin, chicken breast, salmon, and shrimp. Ask for shredded lettuce in place of rice and pile on the vegetables. A small serving of beans will give you slow-burning carbs and fiber. Create your own salads are great choices. You are the one in total control of what goes on your plate. Begin with a bed of lettuce, add protein such as pork or chicken, top with pico de gallo, beans and a time amount of olives, guacamole, and cheese.

Quick Service/Casual Dining Restaurants

Large menus with endless choices seem like a conscious eater's undoing. You need to know what to look for. Salads with a source of protein is always a good choice. Don't use any more than two tablespoons of dressing. Keep high-calorie toppings like avocado, seeds, nuts, and cheese small. Have breakfast for dinner like a veggie omelet with just a bit of cheese. Skip the fries and toast and opt for a side of fruit or turkey bacon. Other choices include broiled or baked chicken or seafood with a side of vegetables, chili, half of a wrap filled with veggies and protein, or broth-based or bean soup. Ask for gravy or sauce to be served on the side or leave them off completely.

Chinese and Thai

With Chinese and Thai cuisine it is easy to make unhealthy or healthy choices. There are huge amounts of calories, carbs, and fats on their menus. Stay away from noodle dishes such as lo mein, dumplings, and pad thai. The same goes for battered, and fried seafood or meat dishes like sweet and sour pork, General Tso's chicken. Steer clear of tempura anything, spring rolls, egg rolls, and fried rice. If it says crispy or crunchy, it has been fried.

Choices that will be pleasing to your taste buds are seafood, shrimp skewers, grilled chicken, hot and sour soups, chicken lettuce wraps, and Thai summer rolls. A couple of appetizers can make a meal. If you want a complete meal, choose stir-fried vegetables and protein. Remember eggplant, tofu, shrimp with vegetables, beef and broccoli. White sauces are lighter in oil. Ask if you have any questions.

Japanese

The main tip to incorporate is to eat with chopsticks. They will slow down your eating, and this results in fewer calories. Stick with entrees such as teriyaki shrimp, chicken, or tofu with vegetables. Stay away from rice.

Indian

Ordering a dish that lists its ingredients will help you make choices. If you are eating at a buffet, here are some tips to navigate around the restaurant.

Avoid anything that is covered in dough or batter and is deep-fried. Don't choose padoka and samosas; these are high in carbs, fat, and calories. Stay away from ghee based sauces like dum aloo, or butter chicken. Skip the naan.

Anything with vegetables and lean meats or seafood like lamb kabobs, chicken, or prawn. Yellow lentils are prepared in less fat.

Chicken or BBQ Restaurants

Stay away from high-fat meats, anything deep-fried, high in calories, and high carb. If you can get grilled chicken, go for it. If not, choose chicken and remove the skin. If ribs are your favorite, they are protein but are high in calories and fat. Boiling them will cook off most of the fat. Ask your server for the leanest choice. If they ask what seasoning, a dry-rub has less sugar and calories than barbecue sauce. Choose a side carefully like salad, green beans, mushrooms, or asparagus. Coleslaw or half an ear of corn would be okay.

Rest Stops and Convenience Stores

Some stores will have a deli where you can get some low-fat cheese, lean ham, or turkey breast. If they only have pre-made sandwiches, take off the bread and just eat the insides. Check the refrigerator section for low-fat milk, part-skim cheese sticks, Greek yogurt, or hard-boiled eggs. Non-perishable choices are protein bars, trail mix, seeds, and nuts. Check the label for sugar grams when choosing trail mix, bars, and yogurts.

Coffee Shops

If your favorites here end in -cino or -atta, you are about to have your day ruined. These specialty drinks are liquid calorie bombs. They have no place in a post-surgery diet. Even the low-fat, skinny, or light versions need to be avoided. Forget their baked goods since there isn't anything like a high-protein, low-carb doughnut. Better choices would be tea, plain iced or hot coffee, unsweetened latte with low-fat milk. Add milk and your favorite no-calorie sweeteners or flavor it with vanilla, lemon, and cinnamon. If you need a snack or breakfast look for protein snack packs, roasted nuts, thin bread or wraps, or yogurt.

Vending machines

You haven't eaten, and you need a snack the only thing available is something from the vending machine. Look for roasted white cheddar popcorn, sunflower seeds, or roasted nuts. The small size and combination of fat, protein, and fiber should keep you full enough to make it to a protein-based meal.

What to do Through the Holidays?

Stick with your nutrition plan if you can. Be sure you are getting enough protein and fluids. You can incorporate your favorite holiday dishes into your menu.

Choose desserts and foods that are low in sugar. Stay away from sugar intake to prevent dumping syndrome and weight gain. Adapt your holiday desserts with Stevia instead of sugar.

Portion control. Portion out the meal before you sit down at the table. If you use small plates and utensils, it will keep you on track. Use a salad plate in place of a dinner plate. This will decrease your intake without you realizing it.

Sit, eat slowly and enjoy your food. Remember to sit and watch what and how much you are eating. Put the fork down between bites. This will help you slow down the food intake. Focus on the food you are eating. Stick to your meal plan and new habits.

Stop when you are full. Stop eating when you feel full. Save any leftovers for a snack to make sure you are getting the right protein intake. Eat slow.

Fluids, fluids, fluids. Make sure you are staying hydrated. Make sure you are consuming 64 ounces of water each day. Try sugar-free cider or hot cocoa.

Stay away from temptations. Do you have leftovers? If you are facing temptations and can't stick to portion sizes, throw them away or give them to family or friends.

Just because you are exercising it doesn't mean you can eat more. Your exercise and nutrition plan has to work together to achieve your goals after surgery. You shouldn't have to exercise more just to cover up extra calories you are consuming.

Got the holiday blues? This time of year can cause many people to become stressed and depressed. If you have a counselor, schedule an appointment to work through your problems. Surround yourself with people that support and lift you up. Count your blessings.

Focus on activities that don't require foods. See the lights, go ice skating, browse the department store windows. Check out a show, go skiing. Donate clothes, toys, and gifts to local shelters or charities. Don't forget all the animals that need supplies and food at the local shelters.

Exercise

After gastric bypass surgery, you will be preparing for a new life. A life that is full of regular exercise and healthy eating choices. This results in an improved you. There are several different exercises that you are able to do while recovering from surgery. As you heal, you are going to be able to add more challenging exercises to your routine.

It all depends on your level of fitness before you had surgery. Your doctor will tell you how much and when you will be able to start working out. Doctors normally recommend that you don't engage in physical activities other than walking during the first three months after surgery. Here are some post gastric bypass surgery exercises that you can use and then modify with each stage of recovery:

Low Impact – Two to Four Weeks After

The first few weeks after surgery you will be focusing on your recovery. Once you have your doctor's permission, you will start doing low impact exercise like:

- Walking – This is the simplest thing you can do, but it is the most effective way to start building stamina. Begin by walking for just ten minutes two times a day. Gradually work up until you can walk for 30 minutes easily.

Sitting Exercises

- Arm rotations – Raise your arms straight out at shoulder level. Move them in little circular rotations backward and forward.

- Shoulder rolls – This is very easy. You will roll the shoulders forward and backward.

- Leg lifts – While you are sitting, lift the legs as if you are marching.

Cardio and Aerobics – One to Three Months After

By the first month after surgery, you should be healed enough to start some challenging exercises. Be sure to go at your pace and stay in contact with you surgeon if you have problems. Here are some low impact exercises:

- Water aerobics – This is very effective and has the lowest injury rate. Most gyms offer water aerobics classes that you can join, or just swim a few laps each day.

- Cycling – Riding a bike is a wonderful exercise for the joints. You can attend cycling classes or ride around your neighborhood. Ride for about 30 minutes each day, five days a week.

Strength Training – Four Months After

Strength training is needed to help lose weight after surgery. Strength training will allow you to build muscle, improve balance, and burn calories. Get your doctor's permission and begin strength training three times a week. Here are some beginner strength training exercises:

- Yoga – This is a mix of relaxation and strength training. You can get a yoga DVD to do in your own home. You can also find places that offer classes in your neighborhood.
- Lunges and Squats – Both are effective exercises that can help your leg muscles. Getting these muscles stronger will help you do longer endurance exercises.

Begin slow. There is a difference between sharp pain and sore muscles. If something feels off, stop and contact your doctor. Your surgeon will recommend the exercises for you and see that you are on the right track.

You are ready to celebrate your new, healthy lifestyle. All of the hard work will result in much happier and healthier years to come.

Conclusion

Thank for making it through to the end of *Gastric Bypass Diet Guide.* Let's hope it was informative and able to provide you with all of the tools you need to achieve your goals.

The next step is to take what you have learned here to help you make the decision of whether or not gastric bypass surgery is right for you.

Finally, if you found this book useful in any way, a review on Amazon is always appreciated!

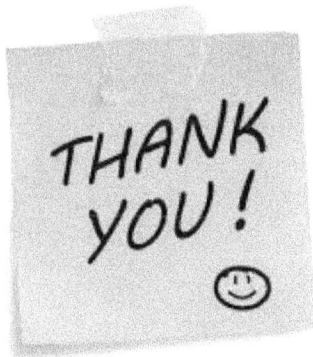

Gastric Bypass Recipes

80+ Simple Recipes for the First Stage After Gastric Bypass Surgery

Bonus:
FREE Report Reveals The Secrets To Lose Weight

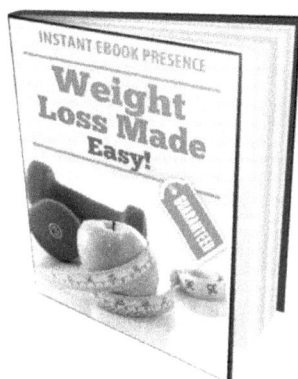

Weight loss doesn't happen from dieting only. Diets are short term solutions to shed extra weight. Diets do not work in the long term because people hate being on a diet (it's ok, you can admit that here). The only long term solution for permanent weight loss is to create new eating habits. This doesn't mean that chocolate will never pass your lips again, but it does mean looking after yourself and watching what you eat...

You can lose weight when you have the right reasons and motivation, and a part of this guide is to help you to find the motivation you need to change your weight...

Go Here to Get This Guid For FREE

http://www.sportsforsoul.com/weight-loss-2/

Table of Contents

Introduction

Congratulations on downloading your personal copy of *Gastric Bypass Recipes.* Thank you for doing so.

The following chapters will provide you with information to help you through the first stages after you have your gastric bypass surgery

You will discover how important it is to control what and how you eat so that you don't experience any adverse effects.

There are plenty of books on this subject on the market, thanks again for choosing this one! Every effort was made to ensure it is full of as much useful information as possible. Please enjoy!

Congratulations on downloading your personal copy of *Gastric Bypass Recipes*. Thank you for doing so.

Guide for the After Surgery

People who have undergone gastric bypass surgery will have to follow a specific diet, especially right after their operation. They will gradually learn how to they can and can't eat so that they don't experience any discomfort.

Gastric bypass is only one form of weight-loss surgeries that are currently performed. The operation has undergone many changes since it was first used. The gastric bypass that is performed today is known as Roux-en-Y. Do not confuse gastric bypass with other weight-loss operations such as biliopancreatic diversion with duodenal switch as this kind of surgery is a lot more aggressive. When you have the surgery, you will talk with your dietitian or doctor, and they will inform on how you should eat after your operation, and they will explain the foods that can eat and how much. If you follow the plan they out for you closely, then you will safely lose weight.

To help get you started, and in the right mindset, let's look at what your doctor is likely to tell you.

There are many reasons why a person starts following a gastric bypass diet. These include:

- To keep from experiencing complications or side effect after the surgery
- To avoid gaining weight and to help them lose weight
- To help you become used to eating smaller portions of food that your stomach will be able to safely and comfortably digest
- To give the stomach time to heal so that the food you eat won't stretch it out

The diet recommendations that you receive after surgery typically vary depending on who does your surgery, where you get it done, and your situation. You will first go through different stages right after your surgery before you enter into your gastric bypass diet. The movement through these stages will depend on how well you heal and can adjust to the new eating patterns. You will likely be able to eat regular foods three months after the surgery.

After you have your surgery, you have to make sure that you drink plenty of fluids so that you don't become dehydrated, and to pay attention to when you feel full or hungry.

On the first day or two after your surgery, you will only get to drink clear liquids. You will have to sip slowly, and you can only drink two to three ounces at a time. After you can handle clear liquids, you will be able to start having other types of liquids, like low-fat or skim milk.

During stage one you can have:

- Sugar-free popsicles or gelatin
- Strained cream soup
- 1% or skim milk
- Decaf coffee or tea
- Unsweetened juice broth

After your system has become used to only liquids for a couple of days, you can start eating pureed and strained foods. You should only consume foods that are the consistency of a thick liquid or smooth paste, without the presence of solid pieces in the mix.

When you are picking foods to puree it best to pick foods that blend well, like:

- Cottage cheese
- Cooked vegetables and soft fruits
- Eggs
- Fish
- Beans
- Lean ground meats

Use these liquids to blend with:

- Broth
- No sugar added juice
- Skim milk
- Water

It's also important to remember that you shouldn't drink and eat at the same time. You need to wait 30 minutes after you eat before you drink anything. Keep in mind that during this time that your digestive system can still be sensitive to certain foods like dairy or spicy foods. If you want to start eating these foods at this time, slowly add them back into your diet with small amounts.

Once you receive your doctor's okay, after a few weeks on pureed foods, you can start to add in soft foods. These should be in the form of tender, small, and easily chewed pieces. During this time, you can start adding:

- Cooked vegetables, without the skin
- Canned or soft fresh fruit, with the seeds and skin, removed
- Finely diced or ground meats

After you have been on this diet for about eight weeks, you will be able to slowly add in firmer foods, but you need to make sure that they are diced or chopped. Make sure you slowly add in regular foods to find out what you can tolerate. You may discover that you still have a hard time with spicy foods, or with foods that have a crunchy texture.

Even once you reach this stage, there are certain foods that you shouldn't eat because they can cause symptoms like vomiting, nausea, or pain. You should avoid:

- Breads
- Fried foods
- Meats with gristle or tough meats

- Fibrous or stringy vegetables, like cabbage, corn, broccoli, or celery
- Granola
- Carbonated beverages
- Dried fruits
- Popcorn
- Seeds and nuts

After some time, you can try to add these foods back into your diet with your doctor's guidance.

Once you hit three to four months after your surgery, you will be able to begin eating a healthy and normal diet, depending on what your situation is, and depending on the foods that you can't tolerate. It's also possible that foods you found irritating right after your surgery, you can now eat after you stomach has healed.

To make sure that you receive enough minerals and vitamins, and to keep yourself on track for your weight-loss goals, at every stage of your diet, make sure you:

- Drink and eat slowly. When you eat or drink too fast, you may experience dumping syndrome. This is when liquids and foods enter into your small intestine quickly and in a larger amount than normal, which causes sweating, dizziness, vomiting, nausea, and soon, diarrhea. To prevent this from happening, eat liquids and foods low in sugar and fat, drink and eat slowly, and then wait 30 to 45 minutes after every meal to drink. Eating your meal should take at least 30 minutes, and it should take 30 to 60 minutes to drink a cup of liquid.

- Eat small meals. As your diet progresses, you should eat many small meals throughout the day, and slowly sip liquids. You may even want to start with six small meals a day at first, move towards four meals, and then return to a regular diet of three meals each day. Every meal should have a half-cup to a cup of food. You should only eat the recommended serving, and make sure to stop eating before you are full.

- Have your liquids between meals. You should drink six to eight cups of fluids each day so that you don't become dehydrated. If you drink liquids with your meals, you will likely feel pain, nausea, and sometimes vomiting, along with the dumping syndrome. If you drink too much around the time of your meal, you may feel too full and can prevent you from eating foods that are nutrient-rich.

- Thoroughly chew your food. The opening that the surgeon created that leads from the stomach to the intestine is tiny, and big pieces of foods may block this opening. Blockages will prevent food from leaving the stomach and will lead to abdominal pain, vomiting, and nausea. Eat small bites, and completely chew them before you swallow. If you are unable to thoroughly chew the food, then do not swallow it.

- Eat foods high in protein. Right after your surgery, eating high-protein foods will help you to heal. Low-fat, high-protein choices should stay as a good long-term diet choice after surgery. Add in lean cuts of beans, fish, pork, chicken, or beef. Low-fat yogurts, cottage cheese, and cheese are also good sources of protein.

- Keep away from foods that are high in sugar and fat. After you have your surgery, it can be hard on the digestive system to tolerate foods that contain a lot of sugars and fat. Keep away from foods like candy bars, fried foods, and ice cream because they are high in fat. Choose sugar-free options like dairy products and soft drinks.

- Introduce foods one at a time. There will be certain foods that you eat after surgery that can cause vomiting, pain, nausea, or can block the opening to your stomach. It will vary from person to person as to what foods they will be able to tolerate. Add new foods one at a time, and make sure you completely chew it. If what you eat causes any discomfort, don't continue to eat it. As more time passes, you may find that you can eat it. Liquids and foods that tend to cause discomfort are carbonated beverages, fried foods, raw veggies, bread, and meat.

- Take mineral vitamin supplements. Since a part of your small intestine will be bypassed after surgery, the body will have problems absorbing the need nutrients from your food. You will probably have to take a multivitamin every day for the remainder of your life. You will need to talk with your doctor as to which vitamin is best for you and if there is any need for you to take anything else, like calcium.

Long term weight loss will be the likely result from your gastric bypass surgery. How much you lose will depend on the kind of weight-loss surgery you have and the lifestyle changes that you make. It is even likely that you will be able to lose half, or more, of the excess weight that you need to within two years time.

This diet will help you to recover from your surgery and to transition into a healthy eating routine and to support your goals for weight-loss. If you return to your old unhealthy eating habits after your surgery, you will probably not lose the weight you need to, or you could gain weight back that you have lost.

The biggest problems that you can encounter from a gastric bypass diet come from not following it properly. When you eat too much or consume foods that you shouldn't, you may experience complications. Complications could include:

- Dumping syndrome. This will typically happen if you eat foods that are high in fat or sugar. These foods have a tendency to travel fast through the stomach pouch and will dump into the intestine. When you experience dumping syndrome, it is accompanied by sweating, dizziness, vomiting, nausea, and diarrhea.

- Dehydration. Since you can't drink fluids along with your meals, people may experience dehydration. To prevent the dehydration, you should sip on 48 to 64 ounces of water each day and other types of low-calorie drinks.

- Vomiting and nausea. When you eat too fast, too much, or don't thoroughly chew your food, you may experience vomiting and nausea after your meals.

- Constipation. When you don't keep a regular eating schedule, don't consume enough fiber, or you don't exercise, you might end up becoming constipated.

- Stomach pouch opening becomes blocked. It's completely possible that food becomes lodged in the opening of your stomach, even if you are extremely careful about following your diet. Symptoms of having a blocked stomach are an abdominal pain, nausea, and vomiting. If you suffer from these symptoms for more than a couple of days, call your doctor.

- Failure to lose weight or weight gain. If you start to gain weight after your surgery, or you don't lose the weight you need to, you may not be eating the right food or consuming too many calories. Speak with your dietitian or doctor to make the best changes for you.

Immediately After Surgery Diet

There are three basic parts of your after surgery diet, no matter which weight-loss surgery you chose to have. In all of them, the first will be fluids, and this will likely be the most challenging. Most people will go home still feeling tired, uncomfortable, and clutching onto their hospital guidelines, and then find themselves wondering in the kitchen unsure of what they should drink or eat.

The first and most important thing is to follow what your bariatric team and surgeon have told you. There will be some surgeons that recommend consuming only clear fluids at first and then adding full fluids during the first few days after surgery; some will have you to continue fluids for a full four weeks after surgery. This is to help minimize digestion, lessen solid waste production, and to ensure maximum healing for the gastrointestinal system.

Clear liquids, the kind you can see through, are the first thing you can start consuming. You should only sip them slowly and never gulp them. You should consume enough so that you stay hydrated, which means you should probably keep a liquid beside you at all times. Make sure that some of these liquids have nutritional qualities so that you receive some nourishment.

Below I will list some of the most common and best choices for liquids, and you will eventually find your favorites. When you first start drinking them, they will likely taste strange, maybe too sweet, so add water or ice to help dilute them so that they have a more acceptable flavor. Variety will likely help during this phase so that you don't end up becoming bored. There may only be a few choices, but it's for the best. These liquids help to maximize your healing process, and you should only move to the next stage when your doctor tells you to.

Generally, you should aim for 2.5 to 3.5 liters of fluid each day. It may seem hard at first to achieve this, but at least try. Spread your drinks out evenly. Everybody will have a different fluid need, and the best way to know if you hydrated is by looking at your urine's color. If your output is pale in color, then you are well hydrated. If it is darker, like straw-colored, or there is only a little bit of urine, you should drink more.

Fluid portion size is recommended to be around six or seven ounces, and in your first few days, this is going to sound like a lot. You should consume each serving about an hour apart. You should also never consume fizzy drinks.

Clear fluid choices include:

- Whey protein isolate fruit drink, such as Syntrax Nectar, mixed with water – this is also good for consuming protein within the early stages

- Vegetable, chicken, or beef broth, bouillon, or consommé, or clear soup

- Sugar-free jelly

- Sugar-free ice pops
- 'Salty' drinks that are diluted in hot water
- Sugar-free or no-sugar-added cordials and squashes
- Coffee, warm and decaffeinated
- Tea, warm and herbal or fruit teas
- Water

It may seem like a long time, but you will eventually move into full liquids, which give you more variety and nutrition. This is an important part because this will prepare your stomach for more solid foods. This stage may last for only a couple of days, or several weeks, it will depend on your surgery and doctor. Follow your surgeon's time line.

Full liquids are the type of foods that are pourable and smooth. Mix and match these liquids with the clear liquids to keep hydrated. The way they taste to you may still be a little strange, so you'll need to experiment, but variety is still important so that you can moves sensibly through this and prepare the body for what's to come. It will get better as each day goes by, and you will develop good habits during this stage and reap those effects better.

Full liquid choices:

- Lightly set egg custards
- Low-sugar and low-fat custards
- Homemade poultry, vegetable, or fish soups, pureed until smooth and then dilute them until they are a runny consistency. You can gradually increase the thickness as you go on.
- Options or Highlight hot chocolate drinks
- Smooth-type cup-a-soups
- Cocoa – made with skim milk
- Homemade smoothies and store bought ones, make sure they are not thick

- Slimfast soups and shakes, but this could end up having too much sugar for bypass patients
- Rice Dream milk
- Oatly, or oat-based drinks
- V8 or tomato juice
- Diluted fruit juice
- Mashed potatoes that are mixed with gravy or broth with the consistency of soup
- Whey protein isolate powder combined with milk or water and frozen into ice cream
- Whey protein isolate drinks
- Smooth cream-style soups, low in fat
- Unsweetened plain yogurt without sugar or fruit added
- Milky chai type tea
- Milk – almond, soy, semi-skim, or skim

Recipes

Mocha Frappuccino

Ingredients

Low-sugar chocolate syrup – optional

Low-fat whipped cream – optional

1 c ice

1 tbsp. cocoa powder

3 to 4 drops liquid sweetener

½ c 0% fat Greek yogurt

¼ c unsweetened almond milk

¼ c brewed coffee

Directions

Put the ice, cocoa, sweetener, yogurt, milk, and coffee into your blender and whizz everything together until it is smooth.

Pour the mixture into a mug or glass and swirl in the chocolate syrup and whipped cream. Enjoy.

Coco-Rita Cocktail

Ingredients

2 tbsps. orange juice, fresh

4 tbsps. coconut water

2 tbsps. birch syrup – or favorite sugar-free syrup

5 tbsps. lime juice, fresh

Rock salt – garnish

Lime wedge

Directions

Pick your favorite martini glass, run the lime wedge around the rim and dip it into the rock salt.

Shake the orange juice, coconut water, syrup, and lime juice vigorously together.

Strain the drink into your glass and enjoy.

5-A-Day Smoothie

Ingredients

2/3 c orange juice, fresh

¼ avocado, chopped and peeled

5 tbsps. low-fat coconut milk

Handful spinach leaves

1 dessert pear

1 apple

Directions

Remove the cores from the pear and apple, and slice them into small pieces.

In your blender, add the orange juice, avocado, coconut milk, spinach, pear, and apple. Pulse the mixture together until it is well blended.

Pour the mixture into a glass and enjoy.

Curry Root Soup

Ingredients

Mint leaves, Greek yogurt, and mango chutney for garnish — optional
Squeeze lemon juice
5 c vegetable stock
1 to 2 tsp curry powder
Pepper
2 crushed garlic cloves
Salt
1 lb. carrots, chopped and peeled
1 lb. rutabaga and swede, chopped and peeled
2 leeks, sliced
1 onion, chopped and peeled
Low-fat cooking spray or a little oil

Directions

Place the cooking spray or oil in your skillet and let it warm up. Place the carrots, rutabaga or swede, leeks, and onion in the skillet and sprinkle with the pepper and salt. Let this gently cook for 30 minutes. Give it a stir now and then. Add a touch of water or oil if it looks like it becomes dry. You want the veggies to soften, but their colors should change too much.

Mix in the curry powder and garlic and let this mixture cook for a couple of minutes.

Pour in the stock and allow the mixture to boil. Turn the heat down and let the mixture simmer for about 15 minutes.

In small batches, place the soup in your blender and mix until it is completely thick and smooth. You can use an immersion blender if available. Blend everything in the pot and mix until smooth.

Place everything back in the pan, add the lemon juice. Taste and adjust the flavorings as you need. Serve in a mug or a bowl.

Pumpkin Pie Shake

Ingredients

½ c ice

1 tbsp. pecans

½ tsp cinnamon

1 c nut milk

1 scoop pumpkin pie protein milkshake

Directions

Using a blender, mix all of the ingredients listed above. Blend until you get a smooth consistency. Then, pour the mixture into a glass and enjoy.

Oatmeal Cookie Shake

Ingredients

Squirt low-fat cream, nuts, and cinnamon for garnish – optional

Ice – optional

¼ tsp vanilla

1 scoop vanilla whey protein powder

1 tbsp. oatmeal

½ tsp cinnamon

1 c low-fat nut milk

Directions

Put the ice, vanilla, oatmeal, cinnamon, milk, and protein powder into your blender and pulse a few times until smooth.

Place the mixture into a glass and serve with some nuts, cinnamon, and low-fat cream.

Apple Strudel Shake

Ingredients

Drizzle of sugar-free syrup and squirt of low-fat cream – option

1 scoop vanilla whey protein powder

1 tsp raisins – optional

¼ tsp cinnamon

3 tbsps. unsweetened applesauce

1 c low-fat nut milk

Directions

Put the cinnamon, applesauce, milk, protein powder, and the raisins if you want to use them, into your blender and pulse a few times until mixed.

Place the mixture into a glass and top with sugar-free syrup and low-fat cream, and enjoy.

Berkshire Iced Tea

Ingredients

Mint sprig and lemon slice for garnish
Ice
1 tbsp. rum – optional
1 tbsp. vodka – optional
¼ c 100% grapefruit juice
1 c boiling water
Ginger and lemon flavored tea bag

Directions

Put the tea bag into the water and let the mixture steep for at least five minutes. Take the tea bag out of the water and discard in. Let the mixture cool.

Once everything is cool, add in the grapefruits juice, if you are still in the first stages after surgery, or you can add in the run and vodka if you have been cleared to drink alcohol.

Place into a glass full of ice and garnish with mint sprig and lemon slice.

Fro-Yo Popsicles

Ingredients

2 c strawberries, hulled
2 c Greek yogurt, full-fat – use fat-free if you want or need to, but the full-fat makes for a firmer texture

Directions

Put both of the above ingredients into your blender and puree them together until they are completely smooth.

Spoon this mixture into popsicle molds, or plastic cups with sticks, and place them in the freezer for at least four to six hours, or overnight for the best results

Unmold the popsicles and enjoy.

Cinnamon Spice Shake

Ingredients

1 scoop protein powder – cinnamon bun flavored, or vanilla with a teaspoon of cinnamon

¼ c applesauce, unsweetened

1 c unsweetened almond milk or low-fat skim milk

Directions

Place the protein powder, with or without the cinnamon, applesauce, and milk into your blender and pulse a few times until mixed.

Pour the mixture into a glass and top with a dusting of cinnamon.

Banana Bomb

Ingredients

½ banana, frozen

2 scoops vanilla protein powder

4 oz. almond milk, unsweetened

4 oz. Greek yogurt, fat-free

Directions

Blend all the ingredients using a blender. Blend until you get a smooth consistency.

Dispense the mixture into your favorite glass and top with some pistachios and banana slices if desired.

Frappuccino with Protein

Ingredients

No-cal sweetener – optional

1 ½ c crushed ice

¼ tsp cinnamon

1 scoop vanilla protein powder

½ c vanilla almond milk, unsweetened

3 tbsps. hot water

1 ½ tsp coffee granules, instant

Directions

Stir the water and the coffee granules together until they are fully dissolved. Place the sweetener, ice, cinnamon, protein powder, milk, and coffee into your blender.

Set the blender to ice speed and mix until smooth. You may end up having to press puree a few times, or stir it depending on how your blender works. As you blend the mixture it will become frothier, so mix until it gets to the consistency that you like.

Place the mixture into a glass, top with some nonfat cream if you want, and enjoy.

Jello Cups

Ingredients

Mint sprig and low-fat whipped cream for garnish – optional

1 c fat-free Greek yogurt

1 ¼ c raspberries

1 oz. packet sugar-free jello crystals

Directions

Mix the jello crystals into 3 ¾ cups of boiling water and mix until they have dissolved. Let the mixture cool, but make sure it doesn't set.

Once it is cold, mix in the yogurt and beat until it is combined.

Spread the raspberries into four serving cups. Place the prepared jello over the berries and place in the refrigerator until it has set up.

Serve with a mint sprig and whipped cream if you want.

Egg Nog

Ingredients

2 bananas

Couple drops rum extract

3 eggs, separated

1 tsp nutmeg

Vanilla pod

2 cinnamon sticks

1 ¾ c milk, skim

Directions

Put the nutmeg, seeds from the vanilla pot, cinnamon stick, and milk in a pot. Let the mixture come up to a boil. Let the mixture cool and completely chill. Once it is chilled strain the milk mixture.

Put the yolks into a blender, rum extract, and bananas. Puree the mixture together until smooth. Pour the milk mixture into the blender and combine. It's ready to enjoy, or you can place it in the fridge until you need it, up to 48 hours.

Once ready to drink, whisk up the egg whites until they form stiff peaks. Mix this into the milk mixture. Place into a glass and top with a dusting of nutmeg if you want.

California Prune

Ingredients

1 tbsps. no-sugar added peanut butter

1 tsp wheat germ

1 c berry fruits – canned, fresh, or frozen

2/3 c milk, skim

2/3 California prune juice

1 banana

Directions

Place all of the above ingredients into your blender and mix until it becomes smooth.

Pour half of the smoothie into a serving glass and place the rest in the fridge to have later.

Pumpkin Soup

Ingredients

Pepper

Salt

1 ¾ c vegetable bouillon or stock

2 pcs of ginger, grated

14 oz. coconut milk, reduced fat

1 ½ lb. squash or pumpkin flesh, cubed

2 tsp curry powder

3 crushed garlic cloves

1 large onion or 3 shallots, chopped

Low-fat cooking spray

Directions

Use a generous amount of the low-fat spray to coat a large pan. Let the pan heat up and add the onion or shallot and let it cook for three to four minutes until it has softened up.

Mix in the curry powder, garlic, and ginger and let this cook for another minute. Next, mix in the squash or pumpkin flesh, stock, and coconut milk. Let the mixture come up to a boil, turn down the heat, and then let it simmer for 10 to 12 minutes. The squash or pumpkin should be tender.

Using an immersion blender, blend up the soup mixture until it is completely smooth. You can use a blender or food processor if immersion blender is unavailable. Add salt and pepper according to your taste, and place back on the heat until hot. Serve with a sprinkling of toasted pumpkin seeds if you can tolerate them.

Carrot and Sweet Potato Soup

Ingredients

Grated carrot, snipped chives, and fat-free yogurt for garnish — optional

Pepper

Salt

6 c vegetable stock

1 tsp cumin

1 in piece ginger, grated

1 lb. carrots, chopped and peeled

2 lb. sweet potato, chopped and peeled

Low-fat cooking spray

Directions

Place a generous amount of the nonstick spray on your pan and let the pan heat up. Add the cumin, ginger, carrots, and sweet potato and let it cook for about ten minutes. Make sure you occasionally stir so that everything begins to brown.

Pour in the stock and then add the pepper and salt according to your taste, let the mixture come to a boil. Place on the lid and let the mixture simmer for around 40 minutes, or until the vegetables turn tender.

Using an immersion blender, blend up the soup mixture until it is completely smooth. If you don't have one, you can add batches of the soup into a regular blender or food processor until smooth. Place back into the pan and let everything heat back up.

Serve the soup with a sprinkle of herbs and some plain yogurt if you would like.

Pumpkin Spice Smoothie

Ingredients

Squirt sugar-free whipped cream – optional
2 scoops espresso protein drink
1 c cold water
¼ tsp vanilla
½ tsp pumpkin pie spice
½ c low-fat milk

Directions

Put the vanilla, pumpkin pie spice, and milk in a shaker. Seal the lid and shake it until it is blended.

Pour in the espresso protein drink and the water. Seal the lid and shake it again until well mixed.

Place the mixture into a serving glass and top with some sugar-free whipped cream if you would like.

Shamrock Smoothie

Ingredients

Mint sprigs, garnish
1 oz. unflavored protein powder – optional
2 tbsps. lime juice, fresh
1 kiwi fruit, sliced and peeled
2 c cantaloupe, cubed and frozen

Directions

Put the protein powder, if you using, lime juice, kiwi, and melon in your blender and mix in up until everything has blended

Split the smoothie between two glasses. Top with some mint sprigs and enjoy.

Ham and Pea Soup

Ingredients

Mint and pea shoots for garnish
Pepper
Salt
2 oz. fresh pea shoots
2 tbsps. chopped mint
¼ c cooked bacon or ham, chopped
4 oz. frozen peas
1 stick celery, chopped
3 ¾ c hot vegetable stock or bouillon
5 to 6 new potatoes, with skins and chopped
2 tbsps. light butter
1 onion, chopped

Directions

Place the butter in a pot and allow it to melt. Mix in the potatoes, celery, and onion and allow this cook for about five more minutes.

Pour in the bouillon or stock and allow it to simmer for another 15 minutes or until the potatoes are fork tender.

Mix in the peas and return it to a simmer and cook for another five minutes.

Remove the pot from the heat and mix in the mint and pea shoots, and then the bacon or ham. Stir everything together.

Mix the soup using an immersion blender. Blend until you get a smooth consistency. As an alternative, you can use a blender or food processor and blend the soup by batch. Dash some pepper and salt according to your taste.

Place back in the pot and let the soup heat back up. Garnish with mint and pea shoots if you would like.

Spiced Carrot and Parsnip Soup

Ingredients

1 tsp cumin seeds, toasted – optional

Pepper

Salt

1 orange, zest, and juice

4 ¼ c hot vegetable bouillon or stock

1 lb. carrots, cubed and peeled

1 tbsp. garam masala

1 to 2 red chilies, chopped and deseeded

1 onion, chopped

Low-fat cooking spray

Directions

Spray a large pot with a generous amount of the nonstick spray. Let the pot heat up and then mix in the chili and onion and allow it to cook for five minutes until they are soft. Mix in the garam masala and let it all cook for another minute.

Mix in a cup of water, stock, carrots, and parsnips. Let the mixture come to boil and place on the lid. Let the mixture simmer for 20 to 25 minutes, or until the veggies have become tender.

Using an immersion blender, mix up the soup until it is smooth. As an alternative, you can use a food processor or blender. Add the pepper, orange juice, salt, and orange zest. Place back in the pot over the heat and let it warm back up. Serve with cumin seeds if you would like.

Carrot, Lentil, and Apple Soup

Ingredients

4 tbsps. cilantro, chopped, for garnish
4 tbsps. Greek yogurt, fat-free, for garnish
Pepper
Salt
1 c coconut milk, light
3 c hot vegetable bouillon
2/3 c split red lentils
1 celery stalk, sliced finely
2 apples, cored, peeled, and chopped
1 lb. carrots, cut and peeled
Low-fat cooking spray
2 tsp cumin seeds
½ tsp chili flakes

Directions

Get a large pot heated and add in the cumin seeds and the chili flakes. Let this dry-fry for a minute, or until you start to smell their aroma and they start to pop. Take out half of the seeds, leaving the rest in the pot.

Add a generous amount of the nonstick spray, and let it heat. Add in the celery, apple, and carrots. Let this mixture cook for around five minutes and then mix in the coconut milk, bouillon or stock, and lentils. Let the mixture come up to a simmer, place on the lid, and let it cook for about 15 minutes. The lentils and carrots should be tender.

Use an immersion blender to puree the mixture until smooth. If you don't have one, place small amounts in a regular blender and mixture it up until all is smooth. Add in pepper and salt to your taste.

Serve the soup with cilantro and some yogurt. Add on some of the reserved spices.

Pumpkin Pepper Soup

Ingredients

1 tbsp. toasted pumpkin seeds

2 tsp fresh chives, chopped

4 tbsps. Greek yogurt, fat-free

Pepper

Salt

5 c strong vegetable stock

1 tsp thyme leaves

4 garlic cloves, crushed and peeled

1 red chili, chopped and deseeded

1 ½ lb. pumpkin, diced and peeled

6 shallots, chopped and peeled

Low-fat cooking spray

4 red peppers, quartered and deseeded

Directions

Your oven should be set to 400.

Put the red peppers, with skin side up, onto a baking sheet and place them in the oven to roast for 20 to 25 minutes, or until the skin has charred up. Take them off the baking sheet and put them in a bowl. Cover the bowl with saran wrap and let the peppers cool. After they are cooled, peel the skins off and keep the fresh flesh.

While the peppers are getting ready, spray your skillet with a cooking spray. As an alternative, you can brush the skillet with butter or cooking oil. Let the skillet heat up and add in the red chili, pumpkin, and shallots. Let them cook for five to ten minutes, or until everything has softened up.

Mix in the thyme and garlic and let it cook for another minute. Pour in the stock and allow the mixture to boil. Turn the heat down and place on the lid, allowing it to simmer for about 15 minutes.

Place the pepper, red peppers, and salt and let it cook for another five minutes.

Finish up the soup by blending it with an immersion blender or a regular blender until completely smooth. Taste the soup and adjust any of the flavorings that you need to. Place the soup back over the heat, and heat it back to hot. Serve the soup with some pumpkin seeds, chives, and yogurt.

Cauliflower Cheese Soup

Ingredients

Grated nutmegs, pepper, and salt for seasoning

1 ½ c grated hard cheese, low-fat

3 ¾ c milk, skim

2 garlic cloves, chopped

1 potato, large

1 head cauliflower, small to medium

Directions

Trim up, wash, and then chop up the cauliflower, getting rid of the rough stalks. Peel the potato and then finely chop.

Put the milk, garlic, potato, and cauliflower in the skillet and let it heat up on low. Let the mixture simmer until the potato pieces have become fork tender. This will take around ten to 12 minutes.

Mix in the nutmegs, pepper, cheese, and salt and use an immersion blender to mix up the soup until smooth. You can also place it in a regular blender and mix until smooth. Make sure it's piping hot before you serve, or serve at room temperature.

Pink Lady Lollies

Ingredients

6 tbsps. Splenda

1 lb. frozen or fresh mixed summer or forest berry fruits

2 apples, pink lady

Directions

Core, peel, and chop up the apples and place them in a pan with four tablespoons of water. Let them cook for about four minutes.

Add in the berries and let it cook for another three minutes.

Take them off the heat and then mix in the sweetener until it has dissolved. Taste the mixture and add more sweetener if you need to.

Mix this up in a blender and strain to get rid of the seeds. Let the mixture cool and place them in popsicle molds. Allow them to freeze overnight until they have firmed up.

Pea and Leek Soup

Ingredients

Leek twists and mint sprigs for garnish – optional

½ lb. soft cheese, fat-free

Pepper

Salt

½ lb. peas, frozen

4 ¼ c vegetable stock or bouillon

1 tsp olive oil

1 tbsp. low-fat spread

20 mint leaves, chopped

2 lettuce hearts, chopped

1 ¼ lb. medium leeks, chopped and trimmed

Directions

Place the oil, spread, mint, lettuce, and leeks in a large skillet. Let this gently warm up until everything starts to soften.

Mix in the bouillon or stock and let it simmer for five minutes. Mix in the pepper, peas, and salt. Let this cook for another five minutes.

Pour this mixture into a blender along with the cheese and mix until smooth. Place back into the skillet and let everything warm together. Do not let this mixture come to a boil.

Serve cold or warm with a garnish of leeks and mint.

Red Thai Pumpkin Soup

Ingredients

Chopped cilantro for garnish – optional

Lime juice

Pepper

Salt

3 tbsps. red Thai curry paste

2 ½ c vegetable stock

1 can pumpkin

1 ¾ c coconut milk, reduced fat

1 tsp chopped lemongrass – optional

1 tbsp. ginger, chopped

1 onion, chopped and peeled

Light cooking spray

Directions

Coat a large skillet with some cooking spray. Mix in the lemongrass, if using, ginger, and onion and let it cook for at least ten minutes, or until everything has softened.

Mix in the pepper, curry paste, salt, stock, pumpkin, and coconut milk, and combine well. Place on the lid and allow the mixture to cook for 15 minutes. Occasionally stir the mixture.

Pour everything into your blender and mix it up until smooth. Place back in the skillet and let everything heat through. Add a little squeeze of lime to the dish and top with some chopped cilantro.

Cheesy Broccoli Soup

Ingredients

Croutons – optional

Pepper

Salt

5.2 oz. dolcelatte cheese

4 1/3 vegetable stock

2 7 oz. packs of broccoli

Bay leaf

1 potato, diced and peeled

2 garlic cloves, crushed

1 onion, chopped

Light cooking spray

Directions

Generously spray a skillet with cooking spray. Place in the onion and cook for five minutes until it has softened, but the color should not change. Stir in the bay leaf, garlic, and potato. Place on the lid and let it cook for another five minutes. Stir occasionally until the potatoes have softened.

While that's cooking, chop the broccoli up into small pieces and place them in the skillet along with the stock. Let everything come up to a simmer and continue to cook for around five minutes or until the broccoli becomes tender. Chop up the dolcelatte roughly and mix it into the skillet until it is soft.

Take out the bay leaf. With either a regular blender or an immersion blender, mix up the soup until smooth. Add in pepper and salt to your tasting.

Serve with croutons if you would like.

Turkish Mint Soup

Ingredients

Pepper

Salt

2 1/5 c vegetable stock

Handful mint, chopped

14 oz. lentils

14 oz. tomatoes, chopped

1 garlic clove, crushed

1 onion, chopped

Light cooking spray

Directions

Coat a pan with some of the cooking spray. Place the garlic and onion and let them cook until they have softened around three to five minutes.

Mix in the pepper, stock, salt, entire contents of lentils can, and tomatoes.

Let the mixture boil. Reduce the heat and cover with lid. Let it simmer for another 15 to 20 minutes.

Place the mixture into your blender and mix until it is completely smooth.

Beetroot Smoothie

Ingredients

1 beetroot, cooked

½ c orange juice

½ c pomegranate juice

Directions

Place all of the above ingredients into your blender and whizz it all together.

Strawberry Kiwi Smoothie

Ingredients

½ c low-fat milk

1 banana, sliced

1 kiwi fruit, chopped and peeled

3 strawberries, large

Directions

Process the banana, strawberries, milk, and kiwi together in your blender until it is smooth.

Egg Custard

Ingredients

½ tsp vanilla

4 tbsps. Splenda

4 egg yolks

2 ½ c milk, skim

Directions

Place the milk in a heavy pot and let it come up to a boil.

Using a large bowl, beat the Splenda and yolks together until they are creamy.

Place the milk into the whipped yolks, and beat together until well blended. Rinse out the pot.

Strain the egg mixture through a sieve and put it back into the pot and cook at a low temp. Let it cook while you constantly stir until everything has started to thicken up to where it will coat your spoon and has a heavy cream consistency.

Serve as it is, cold, or with a dusting of nutmeg. You can also add bananas or fruit puree if you are in the stage to handle them.

Chocolate Ice Cream

Ingredients

2 tbsps. hot chocolate powder, low-fat

2/3 c milk, skim

2/3 c custard, low-fat

2 scoops flavorless protein powder

4-4 oz. vanilla and chocolate yogurt

Directions

Combine the chocolate powder, milk, custard, protein powder, and the yogurt.

Place the mixture in the freezer and freeze until it has firmed up. Make sure you check every so often and whisk it up a few times before it is completely hard. This makes sure that it doesn't form large ice crystals. You can use an ice cream maker to freeze it if available.

Let it soften for about 30 minutes before serving.

Mango Smoothie

Ingredients

2/3 c milk, reduced-fat or skim

1 scoop protein powder

½ mango, chopped and peeled

Directions

Place all of the above ingredients in your blender and mix until it is completely smooth.

Banana and Coconut Puree

Ingredients

¼ tsp cinnamon

1 to 2 tbsps. canned coconut milk, low-fat

½ banana, peeled

Directions

Put the bananas in a bowl and mash them up with a fork until it is about smooth.

Place the banana in the microwave and set it for 10 seconds, stir it around, and heat it for another 10 seconds. Continue this until it is warmed through.

Mix in the cinnamon and coconut milk.

This can store in the fridge for one day, or you can freeze it up for three months.

Cheeseburger Soup

Ingredients

16 oz. Velveeta cheese, cubed, or 2 c shredded cheddar
½ tsp pepper
½ tsp salt
2 c milk, skim
¼ c AP flour
3 tbsps. butter
1 lb. ground beef, lean
3 c chicken broth
1 tsp parsley, dried
1 tsp basil, dried
½ c celery, diced
1 c carrots, shredded
1 small onion, chopped
4 small potatoes, diced and peeled

Directions

Put the parsley, basil, celery, carrots, onions, and potatoes in your slow cooker. Add in the broth. Place on the slow cooker lid. Set your cooker to a low heat and set it for six to eight hour, or, if you need it done faster, you can set your cooker to high for four to five hours. The potatoes should be tender.

At around 45 minutes before you plan on enjoying your soup, you should cook the beef and place it into your cooker. Wipe out the skillet you used and melt the butter. Whisk the flour into the butter and let it cook until it becomes browned and bubbly. Stir in your milk, pepper, and salt. Place this into your slow cooker and stir everything together.

Add the cheese, Velveeta or shredded, and stir everything together well. Place the lid on the cooker and let it cook for another 30 minutes. You can enjoy it like this if you can eat solid foods. If you are still in the liquid/pureed phase, take your immersion blender and blend it up until it is smooth.

Buffalo Chicken Dip

Ingredients

1 c mozzarella, reduced-fat

2 c shredded chicken, cooked

2/3 c hot sauce

2 tbsps. ranch dip seasoning – optional spicy flavor

1 c 0% Greek yogurt

10 oz. Neufchatel cream cheese, room temp

Directions

You should place all of the above ingredients into your slow cooker. It is best to use a slow cooker liner in this process as t can make everything a lot easier.

You should set the cooker to low at three to four hours. Make sure you stir it every hour.

Once this is done, make sure that the chicken is shredded and mashed up enough, and that there is enough liquid so that it has a thin consistency.

Cauliflower Cheese Soup

Ingredients

Cilantro – optional

1/8 tsp cayenne

Pepper

Salt

5 ½ oz. sharp white cheddar, grated

4 c chicken broth, plus a little extra if needed

1 head cauliflower, medium, trimmed and cut into small pieces

1 large onion, diced

3 tbsps. butter

Directions

Place the butter into a big pot and let it melt. Mix in the onion and let it cook until it has softened; make sure that you stir often. Place in the cauliflower and let it cook until it starts to brown up. This will likely take about 12 minutes.

Add in a cup of water and the broth and let the mixture come to a boil. Lower the amount of heat and let the mixture continue to cook until the cauliflower until it is tender. This will take around 20 minutes. Let this mixture cool and little.

Place batches of the mixture into a blender and mix it until smooth. Continue doing this until you puree all of the soup. Make sure you are careful because the soup will still be hot.

Place everything back into your big pot, and add in some more water or broth to thin it out a bit if you need to.

Let everything heat through and mix in the cheese, stirring until it has melted completely. Add the pepper, salt, and a little sprinkle of cayenne.

Garnish the soup with cilantro if you would like.

Pureed Pintos

Ingredients

½ c chicken broth

2 cloves garlic, chopped

1 c salsa

1 medium onion, diced

15 oz. pinto beans, rinsed and drained

2 tsp olive oil

Directions

Cook your garlic and onion in a skillet until they have browned up slightly. Place the beans, salsa, and the cooked veggies into your blender. You can also use a food processor if you have. Slowly add in a little chicken broth until it becomes smooth enough for you to eat. Place the mixture into the pan and let it cook until it begins to bubble and bit and heats through.

Soft Eggs with Chives and Ricotta

Ingredients

Olive oil

1 tbsp. chives, chopped

½ c ricotta

½ c milk

2 eggs

Directions

Place the milk and the eggs into a jar. Top with its lid and shake with all your might to scramble the mixture together.

Warm up your skillet and place in the scrambled eggs. Cook and stir the eggs until they become soft-set. Stir the eggs gently now and then.

Once they are just set, mix in the chives and the ricotta. Place the eggs on a plate and serve with a little drizzle of oil if you would like.

Mashed Cauliflower

Ingredients

Pepper

Salt

¼ c chives, chopped

¼ c parmesan, grated

2 c chicken broth

2 small cauliflower heads, cored and cut into florets

Directions

Place the broth and the cauliflower into a pot and let the mixture start to boil. Lower the pots temp and place on the lid. Allow this mixture to continue to cook for around 15 to 20 minutes. The cauliflower needs to be tender, but it should be falling apart.

With a slotted spoon, place the cauliflower into your food processor and mix it until it is completely smooth. Place this into a bowl and mix in the chives and parmesan. Add the pepper and the salt, and mix until it is smooth.

Ricotta Bake

Ingredients

½ c mozzarella, shredded, part skim

½ c marinara sauce

Pepper

Salt

1 tsp Italian seasoning

1 egg, beaten

½ parmesan, grated

8 oz. ricotta cheese, part skim

Directions

Place the seasonings, egg, parmesan, and the ricotta in a bowl and mix it together very well. Pour the mixture into a baking dish that has been coated with cooking spray. Place the marinara sauce over the top and add on the mozzarella cheese. Your oven should be set at 450 and place in the baking dish and let the mixture cook for 20 to 25 minutes. It should become brown and bubbly.

Deviled Egg Salad

Ingredients

Toasted bread – optional

Lettuce – optional

Pepper

Salt

1 tsp garlic powder

1 tsp onion powder

1 tbsp. pickle relish

1 tsp mustard

½ c miracle whip

6 eggs

Directions

Place the six eggs in a pot and fill it up with water. Let the water start to boil and time them to cook for 15 minutes. Once they are done, drain the water, crack the eggs slightly, and let them sit in cold water until cool enough for you to touch.

Peel the cooked eggs and dice them up into smaller bits. Mix the in the miracle whip and all of the other spices until well mixed.

If you want, place this on a slice of toast or lettuce.

Salmon Pate

Ingredients

1/8 tsp pepper

1/8 tsp salt

1 tbsp. lemon juice

½ tsp dill, dried

2 tbsps. 0% fat Greek yogurt

2.5 oz. smoked salmon

Directions

Place the above ingredients, except for the yogurt, into your food processor. Mix everything up until the fish has been diced up finely.

Place the diced fish in a bowl and stir in the yogurt until everything is smooth.

Southwest Bean Dip

Ingredients

1 c pinto beans, drained

1/3 c salsa

¼ c cilantro

½ c Mexican cheese blend

Directions

Place the beans, salsa, and the cilantro in your food processor until it only has a little bit of texture. Pour this mixture into your baking dish and top, or stir the cheese into the bean mixture. Your oven should be set at 350. Let the mixture cook for 25 to 30 minutes.

Cheesecake Protein Pudding

Ingredients

1 pkg cheesecake pudding mix, sugar-free

1 scoop vanilla protein powder – Bari-essentials or Bari-Clear

1 c Greek yogurt

Directions

Place all of the above ingredients into your blender and mix together until completely smooth.

Lemon Ricotta Creme

Ingredients

4 packets Splenda

1 ½ tsp vanilla

1 to 2 tsp lemon extract – or orange

1 lemon, zest – or orange

15 oz. ricotta cheese, low-fat or fat-free

Dircctions

Place everything from the above list into your blender and whirr until they are all smooth and combined.

Refried Bean Soup

Ingredients

16 oz. refried beans

8 oz. ground beef, browned and mixed with ½ packet taco seasoning

1 small onion

1 medium tomato

4 tbsps. green chili peppers

11 oz. Mexican style corn

½ packet taco seasoning

2 c chicken broth

Directions

Place the tomato, onion, beef, and refried beans in your food processor and pulse until they become slightly chopped.

Place this mixture into a pot and add the broth, taco seasoning, and corn and stir together. Let this mixture come up to a boil and cook for about 15 minutes.

Pepperoni Pizza Casserole

Ingredients

½ c mozzarella, shredded

12 pepperoni slices

Pepper

Salt

¼ c mozzarella, shredded

8 pepperoni slices

1 tbsp. butter

2 tbsps. heavy cream

1 head cauliflower

Directions

Clean up the cauliflower and break it into small pieces. Put this in a bowl with the butter and cream. Place this in the microwave, keeping it uncovered, and microwave for ten minutes. Stir the cauliflower so that it gets coated with the cream and butter. Microwave for another six minutes, or until the cauliflower has become tender. Take the tender cauliflower and place it into your food processor as well as a quarter cup of mozzarella, and eight pepperoni slices. Pulse the mixture until it is smooth. Add in pepper and salt according to your taste. You can also adjust the cream and butter to suit your preferences.

Place the mixture into an eight by eight baking dish. Add in a half cup mozzarella and top with the pepperoni. Your oven should be set at 375. Bake the mixture for 20 minutes.

Avocado Potato Puree

Ingredients

Pepper
Salt
2 tsp milk, skim
½ avocado, peeled
2 oz. chicken breast or thigh, boneless and skinless
1 small potato, peeled and chunked

Directions

Cook the chicken and the potato together until the both are cooked through, and the potato is fork tender.

Put this in a blender along with the pepper, salt, milk, and avocado. Mix this up until it smooth. If you need it to be thinner, add in some milk. Adjust the flavors to your taste.

Diner Chicken Salad

Ingredients

¼ tsp pepper
½ tsp salt
2 celery stalks, diced finely
1 tsp mustard
¾ c mayonnaise, light olive oil
2 12oz cans chicken, shredded finely
¼ onion, diced finely

Directions

Put all of this into a bowl and stir it together. Season as you need and adjust the amount of mayo to how creamy you want your chicken salad.

Crab Spread

Ingredients

1 can crab meat, shredded

1 tsp garlic powder

¼ tsp horseradish

1 tbsp. hot mustard

¼ c cheddar cheese, shredded

1 tbsp. Bari-Clear protein powder

¼ c light mayonnaise

½ c cottage cheese, fat-free

¼ c cream cheese, fat-free

Directions

Put the crab meat, cottage cheese, and cream cheese into your food processor and mix it up until it is smooth. Place in a bowl and then stir in all of the remaining ingredients. Place in the microwave for three to five minutes. Allow this to cool for five minutes before you eat it.

Cheese Lasagna

Ingredients

¼ c mozzarella, 2% milk

2 egg whites

¼ tsp basil

¼ tsp oregano

¼ c marinara

¾ c cottage cheese, fat-free

Directions

Combine the basil, oregano, egg whites, and cottage cheese together and put this all in a baking dish. Pour the marinara sauce all over the mixture and then sprinkle on the mozzarella. Your oven should be at 450, and you should cook it for 20 minutes.

Squash Casserole

Ingredients

1 scoop Bari-Clear protein powder

1 tbsp. cheddar cheese, shredded

1 to 2 tsp butter

Pepper

Salt

½ tsp garlic powder

2 tbsps. cream cheese, fat-free

1 can squash with Vidalia

Directions

Put all of the above ingredients into your blender and mix until it is smooth. Pour the mixture into a bowl and let it microwave for 90 seconds.

Parmesan Cauliflower

Ingredients

1 tbsp. bari-clear protein powder

¼ c milk

¼ c parmesan

¼ c mozzarella

¼ tsp pepper

¼ tsp garlic powder

1 tsp salt

1 bag cauliflower florets

Directions

Put the bari-clear, milk, parmesan, pepper, salt, garlic, and cauliflower in your blender and mix until it has become smooth. Place this into a large bowl and add on some mozzarella cheese, and place it in the microwave for 90 seconds.

Enchilada Eggs

Ingredients

Pinch salt

4 eggs

10 oz. enchilada sauce

½ can refried black beans, fat-free

Directions

Place the refried black beans into a pot and let the heat up to a simmer.

In a different skillet, place in the enchilada sauce and let it heat up.

Make four different wells in the enchilada sauce. Gently crack one of the eggs into each of the wells that you just made. Place a covering on the skillet and let the eggs cook for about five minutes if you like soft yolks or if you want them firm.

Place some of the refried beans on a plate and then top with sauce and egg.

Italian Poached Eggs

Ingredients

4 basil leaves, shredded

Pepper

Salt

4 eggs

3 to 4 pieces roasted red pepper, sliced

16 oz. marinara sauce

Directions

Heat up a large skillet and place in the peppers and the marinara sauce.

With a spoon, make a well into the sauce mixture, and repeat this process three more times. Take your eggs, and crack one of them into each of the wells.

Top the eggs with some pepper and salt.

Let this mixture cook for around 12 minutes, or until the eggs have cooked to your desired firmness. You can also cover them if you wish for them to cook slightly faster.

Take the skillet off of the heats and add the torn basil. Scoop out an egg with some sauce and enjoy.

Creamy Deviled Eggs

Ingredients

Dash paprika

Dash pepper

¼ tsp salt

Splash pickle juice

2 tsp mustard

½ c mayonnaise, low-fat

8 eggs

Directions

Place the eggs into a pot and fill it up with water so that the eggs are covered. Set this over heat and allow the water to come up to a boil. Once they are boiling, cook them for 15 minutes. After their done, drain off the water and slightly crack the eggs and cover in cold water.

Once the eggs have cooled to a temp that you can handle, peel them, and slice them in half lengthwise. Carefully take the eggs out and place them in a bowl. Mash up the yolks and stir in the seasonings, mustard, pickle juice, and mayonnaise.

You can use a piping bag for this part if you want otherwise use a spoon to disperse this mixture between the 16 egg halves evenly. Sprinkle the tops with some paprika.

Deviled Egg Dip

Ingredients

3 green onions, sliced and divided

1 tbsp. Dijon mustard

1 tbsp. white vinegar

4 triangles creamy Swiss, Laughing Cow Cheese

½ c mayonnaise, fat-free

8 eggs, hard boiled, divided

Directions

Set one of your cooked eggs aside for use later. Slice all of the eggs along the long side, just like if you were going to make deviled eggs, and take out the yolks, placing them in a food processor. Place in the mustard, vinegar, cheese wedges, mayonnaise, and half of the white parts of the eggs. Mix until the mixture until it is smooth. Scoop this out into a serving bowl.

Chop the rest of the egg whites up and then mix it into the dip as well as 2/3 of the onions.

Take the egg you reserved earlier and chop it up. Add this across the top of the dip with the rest of the green onions. Once you are on regular food, you can serve this with veggies.

Creamy Vegetable Soup

Ingredients

¼ c half and half or coconut milk

3 sprigs thyme – or 1 tsp dried thyme

2 bay leaves

3 c chicken stock

1 tbsp. olive oil

3 cloves garlic, halved and peeled

1 lb. thin skin potatoes

¼ tsp crushed red pepper flakes

Salt

4 celery sticks

1 lb. carrots, peeled

1 large onion

Directions

Chop up the celery, potatoes onion, and carrots into half inch chunks. Set the potatoes to the side by their self away from the other vegetables.

Place oil into a big pot and let it heat up until it shimmers. Add in the celery, onion, and carrots and mix them around in the oil. Add a half teaspoon of salt and the pepper flakes. Let this cook until the vegetables start to sweat, soften up, and the begin smelling sweet. This will take around five to ten minutes.

Mix in the thyme, bay leaves, garlic, and potatoes. Let this mixture cook for another five minutes. If your pot seems dry add in a little bit of oil.

Pour the stock over everything and allow the mixture come up to a boil. Let the heat turn down to a simmer and let it continue to cook until you can easily break into a potato with a fork. This will take about 15 minutes.

To finish up the soup, take it off of the heat. Remove the sprigs of thyme and the bay leaves. If you have an immersion blender, use it up to smooth out the soup, if not, places batches into a regular blender until all of the soup has become smooth.

Mix in the half and half or coconut milk. Taste the soup and adjust any of the flavorings that you need.

Pineapple Dip

Ingredients

1 c plain yogurt, fat-free

4 c pineapple, frozen

Directions

Place both of the above ingredients into your food processor; you can use a blender if you don't have a food processor.

Pulse up the mixture until it is completely smooth and creamy.

Enjoy.

Cauliflower Casserole

Ingredients

¼ c bread crumbs – optional

¾ lb. sharp cheddar cheese

3 c milk

Pepper

1 tsp salt

½ tsp dry mustard

¼ c flour

2 tbsps. butter, divided

4 c cauliflower, steamed

Directions

Once you steam the cauliflower, set it aside. Place three tablespoons of the butter into a pot, allow it to melt and then mix in the seasonings and the flour. Stir in the milk. Mix this until it has thickened up. You should constantly stir to avoid sticking.

Mix in the cheese and pour the mixture over the cauliflower and combine. Sprinkle the bread crumbs if you want to use them and another tablespoon of butter.

Your oven should be set to 375 and place it in and cook for 30 minutes.

This recipe makes a lot of mac and cheese, many servings for bariatric patients as well as the rest of the family. You can also choose to have the recipe as well.

Avocado Tuna Salad

Ingredients

Pepper

Salt

1 lime, juiced

½ red pepper, diced

1 tbsp. pesto

¼ c Greek yogurt, plain

1 can tuna, drained

½ avocado, mashed

Directions

Put all of the above ingredients into a bowl and stir everything together until well mixed. If you are passed the pureed stage, serve with veggies, crackers, or on a sandwich.

Butternut Squash Puree

Ingredients

Pepper

Salt

2 tbsps. coconut oil, butter, or ghee

1 tsp sage, dried – or 1 tbsp. minced sage

1 tbsp. coconut oil or ghee

1 butternut squash

Directions

Your oven should be set at 400 degrees.

Chop up and peel your butternut squash into as even chunks as you can. Coat the squash in the sage and a tablespoon of coconut oil or ghee. Spread the squash out onto a cooking sheet and sprinkle everything with pepper and salt.

Put this in the oven for 30 to 35 minutes, or until the squash has become tender.

Place the roasted squash into a blender, or a food processor if you have one, along with two tablespoons of coconut oil or butter. Mix this up until completely smooth.

Adjust the pepper and salt as you need for your taste.

Street Corn Soup

Ingredients

2 tbsps. + 2 tsp cilantro, divides
1 tsp lime zest
1 tbsp. lime juice
½ c cotija cheese, grated
½ c sour cream
4 c chicken broth
2 garlic cloves, chopped
Pepper, Salt
¼ tsp chili powder
1 c yellow onion, chopped
6 c corn kernels – save 6 cobs for cooking
¼ c olive oil

Directions

Place the oil in a Dutch oven and let it heat up until it begins to shimmer. Place in ½ teaspoon pepper, ½ teaspoon salt, 1/8 teaspoon chili powder, onion, and corn kernels. Cook the mixture, often stirring, until the onions have become soft and the corn begins to brown a little. This should take around ten minutes. Place in the garlic and let cook until it becomes fragrant. Take a cup and a half of this mixture and place it aside. Mix in the broth and the six corn cobs into the Dutch oven. Deglaze the pan to get all the browned bits off the bottom. Allow the mixture to come up to a boil, turn the heat down to a simmer and let it cook for 20 minutes.

Carefully take out the cobs using tongs. Mix in the Cotija and sour cream. Place the mixture, in batches, into a blender and pulse until smooth. You can also use an immersion blender to make it smooth. Place the soup back over the heat. Mix in ¾ of a cup of the reserved corn mixture, two tablespoons of cilantro, and lime juice. Mix in with extra chili powder, pepper, and salt.

Toss the rest of the ¾ cup of reserved corn mixture with two teaspoons of cilantro and lime zest. When serving the soup, add some of the flavored corn mixtures on top and some extra Cotija if you would like.

Banana Custard Pudding

Ingredients

9 bananas, sliced

12 oz. vanilla wafers

1 tsp vanilla extract

¼ c softened butter

4 egg yolks, beaten

7 c milk

¼ c cornstarch

½ c AP flour

2 ½ c sugar

Directions

Mix together the cornstarch, sugar, flour in a bowl.

Place the milk into a big pot and let heat up. You need to bring to 160 F. Slowly add in some of the hot milk into the yolks you beat earlier. Mix the dry ingredients into the tempered eggs and then pour this back into the pot.

As you are constantly stirring, let it cook until it becomes thick and will coat your spoon.

Set the mixture from the heat and mix in the vanilla and butter. Allow the mixture to cool off to room temperature.

Place one-third of your vanilla wafers into the bottom of nine by 13 baking dish. Place half of the banana slices on top of the wafers and then add half of the custard. Top with another third of the wafers, the rest of the bananas and the rest of the custard. Crush up the wafers and sprinkle over the top.

Cauliflower Casserole

Ingredients

Pepper

½ tsp salt

½ c half and half – optional

4 c chicken broth, reduced sodium

2 c water

8 c broccoli, chopped

2 garlic cloves, chopped

1 celery stalk, chopped

1 onion, chopped

1 tbsp. EVOO

1 tbsp. butter

Directions

Place the butter into your Dutch oven and let the butter melt. Mix in the celery and the onion, and cook until they have softened. This will take about four to six minutes. Mix in the thyme and garlic, stirring, until it becomes fragrant.

Mix in the broccoli. Pour in the broth and water and let it come up to a good simmer. Reduce the temp of your heat to maintain the simmer and cook until it is tender. This will take about eight minutes.

In batches, puree your soup in the blender, or use an immersion blender. Mix it back together and add the half and half, if you are using, pepper, and salt.

Pumpkin Cheesecake Pudding

Ingredients

2 tsp pumpkin pie spice

2 scoops vanilla protein powder

1 ½ c milk, skim

2 packs cheesecake pudding mix, sugar-free

1 container cool whip, sugar-free

1 can pumpkin puree – do not get pumpkin pie filling

Directions

Place all of the above ingredients into a bowl. Use a hand mixer and beat it all together until it is all smooth.

Allow the mixture to sit in the fridge for a little while.

Sweet Potato and Beef Puree

Ingredients

1 tbsp. fresh thyme, chopped

2 c beef broth

2 sweet potatoes, chopped and peeled

8 oz. sirloin, cubed

Directions

Place the broth, thyme, sweet potatoes, and beef in a pot and let it all come to a boil. Turn the heat down a bit, so that simmers for 25 to 35 minutes, or until the sweet potatoes are soft and the beef has cooked through. Set this off the heat and allow it to cool a bit.

Place all of this in your blender and mix it up until smooth. Add a little extra broth as needed to thin it out to the consistency that you can eat.

Egg Custard

Ingredients

Grated nutmeg

2 tsp vanilla

2/3 c Splenda

4 eggs

12 oz. evaporated milk

1 c milk

Directions

Your oven should set your oven to 325. Put six custard cups in a large baking pan and place it to the side.

Place the vanilla, Splenda, eggs, evaporated milk, and milk into your blender and press pulse three to four times until it is well mixed and smooth.

Pour this mixture into the six custard cups evenly. Grate a decent amount of nutmeg over the top of every cup.

Pour hot water into the baking pan so that it comes almost halfway up the custard cup sides. Carefully place this into your oven and cook it for 25 to 35 minutes, or until the center set in the center and still slightly jiggly. Your custards should be set before you take them from the oven.

Carefully take the cups out of the water bath and place a towel to cool off.

Jell-O Fluff

Ingredients

1 container Greek yogurt, plain
1 c sugar-free Jell-O, set

Directions

Cook your Jell-O according to the box directions and have it completely set before making this recipe. After it has set, measure a cup of it out and place it in the blender with the Greek yogurt. Mix it up until it is smooth. Place in the fridge or the freezer until it has thickened up, and enjoy.

Instant Pot Custard

Ingredients

Vanilla, to taste
4 tbsps. Splenda
1 ½ c Fairlife whole milk
3 eggs
1 tbsp. sugar

Directions

Sprinkle a tablespoon of sugar into the bottom of a pot that you can fit in your Instant Pot and set it on the heat until the sugar has melted and become browned. Make sure you don't let this burn.

Place all of the remaining ingredients into your blender and mix it up until smooth and carefully place it in the pot.

Place a cup of water into your Instant Pot and place in the trivet. Place the pot with the custard on to the trivet.

Set your pot to cook for five minutes at high pressure and then let the pressure release naturally.

Once done, set the custard in your refrigerator to cool. After it is cooled, gently unmold it and enjoy.

Taco Casserole

Ingredients

2 c Mexican cheese blend, shredded

1 can tomatoes and chiles

1 can refried beans, fat-free

1 can black beans, rinsed and drained

Envelope taco mix

1 garlic clove, minced

1 small onion, diced

1 small squash, diced

1 small zucchini, diced

1 lb. ground meat, lean

Directions

In a skillet that has been coated with some oil, cook the garlic and veggies until they have become soft. Get rid of any excess liquid that the veggies have created, and then place the veggies in a bowl.

Cook the meat until brown, drain off the grease, and then place it in the bowl with the veggies. Add in the tomatoes and canned black beans and stir it all together.

Sprinkle the mixture with taco seasoning and stir to distribute it. Place the mixture in a casserole dish.

Smooth the refried beans over the mixture. It's easier if you heat up the beans before trying to spread them.

Sprinkle over with the cheese. Your oven should be at 350 and bake it for 30 minutes, or until everything has warmed and the cheese is melted.

Allow the mixture to cool for 20 minutes before your serve it.

Chicken and Potato Puree

Ingredients

2 c chicken broth

100% Potato Flakes

Directions

Allow the chicken broth to come to a boil. Set it off the heat and stir in the potato flakes, a tablespoon at a time, until your reach pourable texture. If you add too many flakes, just pour in a little more broth. Add pepper and salt to your liking, and enjoy.

Root Beer Float Ice Cream

Ingredients

½ c Diet Root Bee

1 tbsp. vanilla Torani syrup, sugar-free

2 scoops vanilla protein powder

1 c vanilla soy milk

Directions

Place the soda, syrup, protein powder, and milk in a blender or mixer. Mix it up on high until it is lump free and airy. You can also use a milk frother for this to make it really airy. Place this mixture into an ice cream maker and freeze.

You can eat it as is, or you can freeze it to make it a hard ice cream consistency.

Tortilla Soup

Ingredients

½ c corn tortilla strips
1 c Monterey Jack, grated
1 diced avocado
Salt
4 corn tortillas, diced
14 ½ oz. water
2 14.5 oz. can chicken broth
½ tsp cumin
½ tsp minced garlic
½ bunch cilantro, chopped
2 tomatoes, diced
3 tbsps. oil
1 to 2 serrano chili, minced
1 onion, diced

Directions

In your chosen cooking vessel, preferably a large pot, place in three tablespoons of oil, chilies, and onion, and stir-fry this until you see the onions brown along their edges.

Place in the cumin, garlic, cilantro, and tomatoes and stir-fry this for another three to four minutes.

Add in the corn tortillas, water, and broth. The corn tortillas can be diced, or you can tear them up by hand if you want to. Turn the heat up so that the mixture starts to boil. Turn the heat back down to a maintained simmer and let it cook for 10 to 15 minutes. Once done, set this aside so that it can cool down a little bit.

Using a regular blender or an immersion blender, puree up the mixture until it is smooth.

Place this back in the pot and let it heat back up. Check the taste to adjust the salt level.

Garnish the soup with tortilla strips, cheese, and avocado if you desire.

Chicken Broth

Ingredients

Pepper
Thyme sprig
Parsley sprig
Bay leaf
½ celery stalk
½ carrot
½ onion
3 qts water
3 lb. whole chicken

Directions

Grab yourself a large pot and place all of the above in it. Let the mixture come up to a simmer and cook for an hour to an hour and a half. Reserve the cooked chicken for other recipes and strain out and of the other solids.

Place the strained stock in the refrigerator. The following day, skim the fat off that has risen to the top.

Chicken Puree

Ingredients

1 tsp dried parsley
1 c chicken stock
8 oz. chicken thigh or breast, cubed – skinless and boneless

Directions

Place the above ingredients into a pot and let it come up to a boil. Turn the heat down and let it cook for 15 to 20 minutes. The chicken should be cooked all the way through. Allow the mixture to cool for a few minutes.

Place everything in the pot into your blender and mix it up until it is smooth. If you need to, add more stock to get it creamy.

Baked Potato Soup

Ingredients

Pepper

Salt

½ c sour cream

1 ½ c shredded cheese

3 green onions, sliced

6 potatoes, cubed and peeled

4 c milk

14 c AP flour

5 tbsps. butter, unsalted

1 pack bacon, diced

Directions

Place the cubed and peeled potatoes into water and completely cover them with water to keep them from becoming discolored.

Place the diced bacon into a skillet and cook it until crispy and brown. Place this on a paper towel to get rid of any excess grease.

Melt the butter inside of a big pot. Mix in the flour and cook until it has browned up a bit. Slowly whisk in the milk and allow it to cook while you are stirring so that it starts to thicken. Mix in the potatoes and around half of the onions.

Let this boil for a few minutes, and then turn it down and continue to cook until the potatoes are fork tender. This should take about 15 to 20 minutes. Mix in the pepper, sour cream, salt, and cheese. If the soup has become too thick, add in a bit more milk. For the pureed stage use an immersion blender to make the soup smooth.

You can serve it topped with extra cheese, bacon bits, green onions, and sour cream.

Creamy Shrimp Bisque

Ingredients

Pepper

Salt

½ lb. shrimp, deveined and cleaned

1 c evaporated milk, fat-free

1 bottle clam juice

¼ tsp lemon pepper

1 oz. ham, low-fat

1 tsp garlic, chopped

¼ c onion, chopped

Nonstick spray

1 c cauliflower, steamed

Directions

Add some nonstick spray to a large pot and add in the ham, garlic, and onions and let them cook until soft and brown.

Mix in the shrimp, cauliflower, milk, clam juice, and lemon pepper. Allow this mixture to come up to a boil while stirring often. Allow this to continue to cook until the shrimp become pink.

Mix in the pepper and the salt to your taste.

Place the mixture into your blender and mix it up until smooth.

Peanut Brittle Oatmeal

Ingredients

2 tbsps. Torani brown sugar cinnamon syrup, sugar-free

1 tbsp. sweetener, no-calorie

2 tbsps. PB2

Pinch salt

1 scoop vanilla protein powder

½ c quick oats

Directions

Follow the directions for the brand of quick oats you have. Once it is cooked, mix in all of the other above ingredients. Adjust any of the sweeteners that you need to suit your taste buds.

PB2 Shake

Ingredients

½ c ice

1 tbsp. PB2 powder

1 c milk, skim

1 protein powder – chocolate or classic

Directions

Place all of the above ingredients into your blender. Mix it up until smooth or all of the ice has been crushed up and everything how been combined.

Egg Drop Soup

Ingredients

1 c water
1 egg
1 scoop chicken bouillon granules

Directions

Beat the egg in a bowl until well mixed.

Place the water in a pot and heat it up to boiling. Mix in the chicken bouillon until it has dissolved completely.

Take the egg you beat earlier and fork. As you are stirring the water with the fork, slowly add in the egg so that it forms ribbons of cooked egg. Continue until the egg is mixed in completely. Enjoy.

St. Patrick's Shake

Ingredients

Ice cubes
1 tbsp. pistachio pudding mix, sugar-free
1 Ready to Drink vanilla protein shake – Premier Protein

Directions

Place all of this into your blender and whizz it up until it is smooth.

Yogurt

Ingredients

1 scoop unflavored protein powder
1 c yogurt, favorite fruit flavor – nonfat

Directions

Place all of the above into a bowl and stir together until well mixed. Enjoy.

Sweet Potato Puree

Ingredients

Pepper

Salt

3 large sweet potatoes

Directions

Peel all of the sweet potatoes and then slice them up into two-inch pieces. Place them in a pot and cover them completely with water. Allow the potatoes to boil and cook until they can easily be poked with a fork. This will take about 15 to 20 minutes.

Drain off the water and then puree them in a blender or a food processor if you have one. Mix in some pepper and salt to your taste.

If you want to flavor the sweet potatoes, you can add:

Two tablespoons of maple syrup and butter when you puree the potatoes – Maple Butter

¼ cup of orange juice and milk, two tablespoons of butter, and two teaspoons of ginger when pureeing – Orange Ginger

One tablespoon lime juice and a little bit of cayenne when pureeing – Lime Cayenne

Conclusion

Thank for making it through to the end of *Gastric Bypass Recipes*. Let's hope it was informative and able to provide you with all of the tools you need to achieve your goals.

The next step is to try some of the recipes while you are in your first stages after gastric bypass.

Finally, if you found this book useful in any way, a review on Amazon is always appreciated!

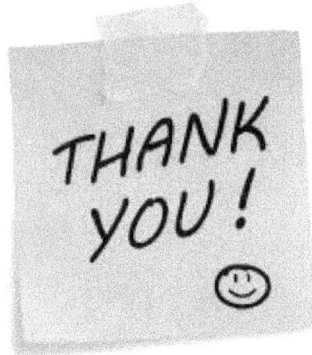

Check Out My Other Books

Below you'll find some of my other popular books that are popular on Amazon and Kindle as well. Simply click on the links below to check them out. Alternatively, you can visit my author page on Amazon to see other work done by me.

CrossFit: Barbell and Dumbbell Exercises for Body Strength

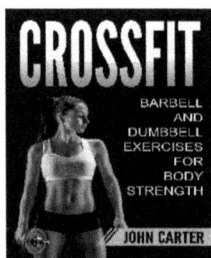

Mediterranean Diet: Step By Step Guide And Proven Recipes For Smart Eating And Weight Loss

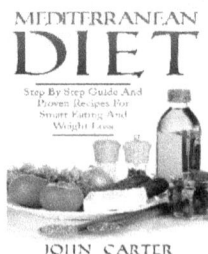

Weight Watchers: Smart Points Cookbook - Step By Step Guide And Proven Recipes For Effective Weight Loss

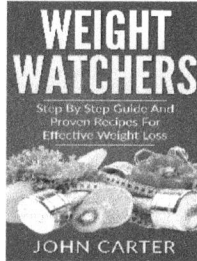

Bodybuilding: Beginners Handbook - Proven Step By Step Guide To Get The Body You Always Dreamed About

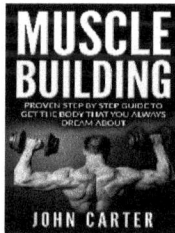

South Beach Diet: Lose Weight and Get Healthy the South Beach Way

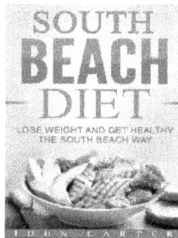

Blood Pressure: Step By Step Guide And Proven Recipes To Lower Your Blood Pressure Without Any Medication

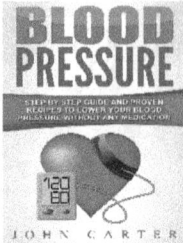

Ketogenic Diet: Step By Step Guide And 70+ Low Carb, Proven Recipes For Rapid Weight Loss

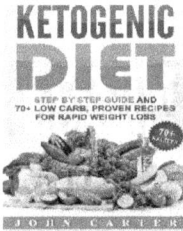

Meal Prep: 65+ Meal Prep Recipes Cookbook – Step By Step Meal Prepping Guide For Rapid Weight Loss

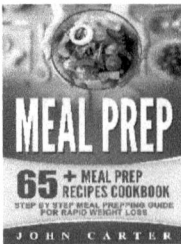

If the links do not work, for whatever reason, you can simply search for these titles on the Amazon website to find them.

www.ingramcontent.com/pod-product-compliance
Lightning Source LLC
Chambersburg PA
CBHW051714020426
42333CB00014B/987